Management of Soft Tissue Trauma

Editor

DONITA DYALRAM

ORAL AND MAXILLOFACIAL SURGERY CLINICS OF NORTH AMERICA

www.oralmaxsurgery.theclinics.com

Consulting Editor
RUI P. FERNANDES

August 2021 • Volume 33 • Number 3

ELSEVIER

1600 John F. Kennedy Boulevard • Suite 1800 • Philadelphia, Pennsylvania, 19103-2899

http://www.oralmaxsurgery.theclinics.com

ORAL AND MAXILLOFACIAL SURGERY CLINICS OF NORTH AMERICA Volume 33, Number 3
August 2021 ISSN 1042-3699, ISBN-13: 978-0-323-80995-5

Editor: John Vassallo; j.vassallo@elsevier.com
Developmental Editor: Jessica Nicole B. Cañaberal

Oral and Maxillofacial Surgery Clinics of North America (ISSN 1042-3699) is published quarterly by Elsevier Inc., 360 Park Avenue South, New York, NY 10010-1710. Months of issue are February, May, August, and November. Business and Editorial Offices: 1600 John F. Kennedy Blvd., Suite 1800, Philadelphia, PA 19103-2899. Periodicals postage paid at New York, NY and additional mailing offices. Subscription prices are $401.00 per year for US individuals, $933.00 per year for US institutions, $100.00 per year for US students/residents, $474.00 per year for Canadian individuals, $984.00 per year for Canadian institutions, $100.00 per year for Canadian students/residents, $525.00 per year for international individuals, $984.00 per year for international institutions and $235.00 per year for international students/residents. To receive student/resident rate, orders must be accompanied by name or affiliated institution, date of term, and the *signature* of program/residency coordinator on institution letterhead. Orders will be billed at individual rate until proof of status is received. Foreign air speed delivery is included in all *Clinics* subscription prices. All prices are subject to change without notice. **POSTMASTER:** Send address changes to *Oral and Maxillofacial Surgery Clinics of North America,* Elsevier Periodicals **Customer Service, 11830 Westline Industrial Drive, St. Louis, MO 63146. Tel: 1-800-654-2452 (U.S. and Canada); 314-447-8871 (outside U.S. and Canada). Fax: 314-447-8029. E-mail: journalscustomerservice-usa@elsevier.com (for print support); journalsonlinesupport-usa@elsevier.com (for online support)**.

Reprints. For copies of 100 or more, of articles in this publication, please contact the Commercial Reprints Department, Elsevier Inc., 360 Park Avenue South, New York, NY 10010-1710. Tel.: 212-633-3874; Fax: 212-633-3820; Email: reprints@elsevier.com.

Oral and Maxillofacial Surgery Clinics of North America is covered in *MEDLINE/PubMed* (*Index Medicus*), *Science Citation Index Expanded (SciSearch®)*, *Journal Citation Reports/Science Edition*, and *Current Contents®/Clinical Medicine*.

Contributors

CONSULTING EDITOR

RUI P. FERNANDES, MD, DMD, FACS, FRCS(Ed)
Clinical Professor and Chief, Division of Head and Neck Surgery, Program Director, Head and Neck Oncologic Surgery and Microvascular Reconstruction Fellowship, Departments of Oral and Maxillofacial Surgery, Neurosurgery, and Orthopaedic Surgery & Rehabilitation, University of Florida Health Science Center, University of Florida College of Medicine, Jacksonville, Florida

EDITOR

DONITA DYALRAM, DDS, MD, FACS
Assistant Professor, Program Director, Oral Maxillofacial Surgery Residency Program, Associate Program Director, Oral-Head and Neck Surgery/Microvascular Surgery, Department of Oral Maxillofacial Surgery, University of Maryland Dental School, Baltimore, Maryland

AUTHORS

MELISSA AMUNDSON, DDS
Attending OMS, Department of Surgery, Trauma Service, Legacy Emanuel Medical Center, Head & Neck Surgical Associates, Portland, Oregon

R. BRYAN BELL, MD, DDS, FACS, FACD
Attending OMS, Department of Surgery, Trauma Service, Legacy Emanuel Medical Center, Consultant, Head & Neck Surgical Associates, Medical Director, Providence Oral, Head and Neck Cancer Program and Clinic, Investigator, The Robert W. Franz Cancer Research Center, Earle A. Chiles Research Institute, Providence Health & Sciences, Portland, Oregon

TUAN BUI, MD, DDS
Director, Oral and Maxillofacial Pathology, Sanford Health, Fargo, North Dakota

NICHOLAS CALLAHAN, MPH, DMD, MD
Assistant Professor, Department of Oral and Maxillofacial Surgery, University of Illinois at Chicago, Assistant Professor, Department of Otolaryngology, Northwestern Memorial Hospital, Chicago, Illinois

ALLEN CHENG, MD, DDS, FACS
Medical Director, Oral/Head and Neck Oncology, Legacy Good Samaritan Cancer Center, Portland, Oregon

ERIC J. DIERKS, MD, DMD, FACS, FACD
Director of Maxillofacial Trauma, Department of Surgery, Trauma Service, Legacy Emanuel Medical Center, Consultant, Head & Neck Surgical Associates, Portland, Oregon

NADIR ELIAS, DMD
Fellow, Advanced Craniomaxillofacial and Trauma Surgery, Legacy Emanuel Medical Center, Portland, Oregon

KYLE S. ETTINGER, MD, DDS
Assistant Professor of Surgery, Section of Head and Neck Oncologic and Reconstructive Surgery, Division of Oral and Maxillofacial

Surgery, Department of Surgery, Mayo Clinic, Rochester, Minnesota

SAVANNAH GELESKO, MD, DDS
Former Resident, Head & Neck Surgical Associates, Portland, Oregon

ASHLEY HOULE, DDS, MD
Resident Physician, Department of Oral and Maxillofacial Surgery, University of Illinois at Chicago, Chicago, Illinois

BABER KHATIB, MD, DDS
Fellow, Advanced Craniomaxillofacial and Trauma Surgery/Head and Neck Oncologic and Microvascular Reconstructive Surgery, Department of Surgery, Legacy Emanuel Medical Center, Providence Portland Hospital, Head & Neck Surgical Associates, Portland, Oregon

DON O. KIKKAWA, MD, FACS
Professor and Chief, Division of Oculofacial Plastic and Reconstructive Surgery, Vice Chair, Department of Ophthalmology, Professor, Division of Plastic Surgery, University of California, San Diego, Department of Surgery, Shiley Eye Institute, La Jolla, California

RODERICK Y. KIM, DDS, MD
Assistant Fellowship Director, Division of Maxillofacial Oncology and Reconstructive Surgery, Department of Oral and Maxillofacial Surgery, John Peter Smith Health Network, Fort Worth, Texas

AUDREY C. KO, MD
Clinical Instructor, Division of Oculofacial Plastic and Reconstructive Surgery, University of California, San Diego, Department of Ophthalmology, Shiley Eye Institute, La Jolla, California

BOBBY S. KORN, MD, PhD, FACS
Associate Professor, Division of Oculofacial Plastic and Reconstructive Surgery, Department of Ophthalmology, Division of Plastic Surgery, University of California, San Diego, Department of Surgery, Shiley Eye Institute, La Jolla, California

MICHAEL R. MARKIEWICZ, DDS, MD, MPH, FACS, FRCD(c), FAAP
Professor and Chair, Department of Oral and Maxillofacial Surgery, William M. Feagans Endowed Chair, Associate Dean for Hospital Affairs, School of Dental Medicine, University at Buffalo, Clinical Professor, Department of Neurosurgery, Division of Pediatric Surgery, Department of Surgery, Jacobs School of Medicine and Biomedical Sciences, Co-Director, Craniofacial Center of Western New York, John Oishei Children's Hospital, Buffalo, New York

MICHAEL MILORO, DMD, MD, FACS
Professor and Department Head, Department of Oral and Maxillofacial Surgery, University of Illinois at Chicago, Chicago, Illinois

JAMES MURPHY, DDS, MD, FACS
Attending, Oral and Maxillofacial Surgery, Cook County Health, Assistant Professor of Plastic Surgery, Rush University Medical Center, Chicago, Illinois

ARTHUR J. NAM, MD, MS
Division of Plastic, Reconstructive and Maxillofacial Surgery, R Adams Cowley Shock Trauma Center, University of Maryland School of Medicine, Baltimore, Maryland

JOHN M. NATHAN, MD, DDS
Senior Resident, Division of Oral and Maxillofacial Surgery, Department of Surgery, Mayo Clinic, Rochester, Minnesota

AMIR NOJOUMI, DMD
Resident, Department of Oral and Maxillofacial Surgery, University of California, San Francisco – Fresno, Community Regional Medical Center, Fresno, California

ASHISH PATEL, MD, DDS
Attending OMS, Department of Surgery, Trauma Service, Legacy Emanuel Medical Center, Consultant, Attending Head and Neck/Microvascular Surgeon, Head & Neck Surgical Associates, Consultant, Providence Oral, Head and Neck Cancer Program and Clinic, Providence Health & Sciences, Portland, Oregon

JOSEPH S. PUTHUMANA, BA
R Adams Cowley Shock Trauma Center, University of Maryland School of Medicine, Baltimore, Maryland

MOHAMMED QAISI, DMD, MD, FACS
Program Director, Cook County Health, Professor of Oral and Maxillofacial Surgery, Midwestern University, Chicago, Illinois

KELLIE R. SATTERFIELD, MD
Physician, Division of Oculofacial Plastic and
Reconstructive Surgery, University of
California, San Diego, Department of
Ophthalmology, Shiley Eye Institute, La Jolla,
California

RAYMOND P. SHUPAK, DMD, MD, MBE
Fellow, Division of Maxillofacial Oncology and
Reconstructive Surgery, Department of Oral
and Maxillofacial Surgery, John Peter Smith
Health Network, Fort Worth, Texas

JAMES THOMAS, MD
Laryngologist, Private Practice,
Voicedoctor.net, Portland, Oregon

FAYETTE C. WILLIAMS, DDS, MD, FACS
Director, Division of Maxillofacial Oncology and
Reconstructive Surgery, Department of Oral

and Maxillofacial Surgery, John Peter Smith
Health Network, Fort Worth, Texas

BRIAN M. WOO, DDS, MD, FACS
Assistant Clinical Professor, Residency
Program Director, Director of Head and Neck
Oncologic Surgery and Microvascular
Reconstruction Fellowship, Department of
Oral and Maxillofacial Surgery, University of
California, San Francisco – Fresno,
Community Regional Medical Center, Fresno,
California

JOSHUA YOON, MD
Division of Plastic, Reconstructive and
Maxillofacial Surgery, R Adams Cowley Shock
Trauma Center, University of Maryland School
of Medicine, Baltimore, Maryland; Department
of Surgery, George Washington University
Hospital, Washington, DC

Contents

Management of Ear Trauma   305

Amir Nojoumi and Brian M. Woo

Facial trauma remains a common reason for visits to the emergency department or urgent care facility. The ear remains susceptible to trauma given its delicate anatomy and position in the maxillofacial region. Understanding the anatomy and recognizing the circumstances regarding the mechanism of injury help dictate treatment. The goals of treatment should remain to restore the physiologic form and function of the ear. Middle ear injuries should also be addressed during the process. Although primary repair remains feasible in most cases, there are instances when delayed and staged reconstruction is necessary to achieve successful results.

Eyelid and Periorbital Soft Tissue Trauma   317

Audrey C. Ko, Kellie R. Satterfield, Bobby S. Korn, and Don O. Kikkawa

Facial trauma often involves injuries to the eyelid and periorbital region. Management of these injuries can be challenging because of the involvement of multiple complex anatomic structures that are in close proximity. Restoration of normal anatomic relationships of the eyelids and periocular structures is essential for optimum functional and aesthetic outcome after trauma. This review provides an overview of the current literature involving soft tissue trauma of the eyelid and periorbital tissue and highlights key steps in patient evaluation and management with various types of injuries.

Management of Nasal Trauma   329

John M. Nathan and Kyle S. Ettinger

Facial trauma can have long-lasting physical and mental consequences. Trauma to the nose is commonly seen in the emergency department. Nasal lacerations account for 7% of all facial lacerations. Thorough examination and documentation including photographs is important for documentation and creating a reconstruction plan. Underlying damage to cartilage or bone must be reconstructed initially or in a delayed fashion to recreate the pretrauma anatomy and function. There are several options for soft tissue nasal reconstruction, including local flaps, skin grafts, pedicle flaps, and free flaps. At present there is no standard of care for postoperative facial trauma wound care.

Management of Salivary Gland Injury   343

Raymond P. Shupak, Fayette C. Williams, and Roderick Y. Kim

Although a rare sequala of soft tissue injury, salivary gland trauma may result in significant morbidity. Salivary gland injury can involve the major as well as the minor glands. Because of the proximity of adjacent vital structures, a thorough history and physical examination are mandatory during patient evaluation. Trauma to the major salivary glands may involve the parenchyma, duct, or neural injury. Treatment requires adherence to primary principles of soft tissue management. Ductal and neural injury should be repaired primarily. Sialocele and fistula are potential complications of repaired and unrepaired salivary gland injury.

Repair of soft tissue trauma to the lips requires careful attention to both function and esthetics. This article outlines basic lip anatomy, goals in managing lip injury, and appropriate workup and ultimate treatment of various types of trauma to the lips.

This article includes updates in the management of mandibular trauma and reconstruction as they relate to maxillomandibular fixation screws, custom hardware, virtual surgical planning, and protocols for use of computer-aided surgery and navigation when managing composite defects from gunshot injuries to the face.

Dogs are the animal most frequently implicated in causing bite injuries to the human face. Dog bite injuries are most prevalent in younger patients. Pasteurella species are commensals of the oral microbiome of dogs and cats and are frequently implicated in infections resulting from dog and cat bite injuries. HIV, hepatitis B, and hepatitis C need to be considered in bites inflicted by humans. All animal bite wounds should be washed out. Most animal bite injuries can be managed in an outpatient setting. Given the cosmetically sensitive nature of the face, bite wounds generally merit suturing, even in delayed presentations.

In the area of craniomaxillofacial trauma, neurosensory disturbances are encountered commonly, especially with regard to the trigeminal and facial nerve systems. This article reviews the specific microanatomy of both cranial nerves V and VII, and evaluates contemporary neurosensory testing, current imaging modalities, and available nerve injury classification systems. In addition, the article proposes treatment paradigms for management of trigeminal and facial nerve injuries, specifically with regard to the craniomaxillofacial trauma setting.

Soft tissue wounds in the scalp are a common occurrence after trauma or resection of a malignancy. The reconstructive surgeon should strive to use the simplest reconstructive technique while optimizing aesthetic outcomes. In general, large defects with infection, previous irradiation (or require postoperative radiation), or with calvarial defects usually require reconstruction with vascularized tissue (ie, micro-vascular free tissue transfer). Smaller defects greater than 3 cm that are not amenable to primary closure can be treated with local flap reconstruction. In all cases, the reconstruction method will need be tailored to the patient's health status, desires, and aesthetic considerations.

Management of Laryngeal Trauma   417

Nadir Elias, James Thomas, and Allen Cheng

The larynx is a complex anatomic structure and a properly functioning larynx is essential for breathing, voice, and swallowing. Laryngeal trauma is often associated with other injuries, including intracranial injuries, penetrating neck injuries, cervical spine fractures, and facial fractures. Although uncommon, laryngotracheal injuries may lead to life-threatening airway emergencies. Because laryngeal injuries are rare, even surgeons with a great deal of experience in managing maxillofacial trauma have limited exposure to management of laryngeal and tracheal injury. This article reviews a protocol for the evaluation, management, and treatment of these injuries in the trauma patient.

ORAL AND MAXILLOFACIAL SURGERY CLINICS OF NORTH AMERICA

SERIES OF RELATED INTEREST

Atlas of the Oral and Maxillofacial Surgery Clinics
www.oralmaxsurgeryatlas.theclinics.com

Dental Clinics
www.dental.theclinics.com

THE CLINICS ARE NOW AVAILABLE ONLINE!
Access your subscription at:
www.theclinics.com

Foreword
Management of Soft Tissue Trauma

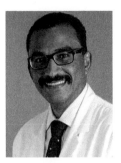

Rui P. Fernandes, MD, DMD, FACS, FRCS(Ed)
Consulting Editor

Trauma management remains one of the cornerstones of the specialty of Oral and Maxillofacial Surgery. Often, the emphasis tends to be on the management of the bony fractures, whereas the management of soft tissue injuries arguably does not receive the same attention. In this issue, we have sought to rectify this neglect. Dr Dyalram has brought together a group of craniomaxillofacial experts to share their approaches toward the management of this important area in craniofacial trauma.

This issue addresses the management of traumatic injuries to the following subsites: scalp, nose, ear, larynx, and lip. In addition, the management of special topics, such as nerve injuries and injuries affecting the salivary gland, has been addressed. Dr Dyalram's choice of authors to tackle these difficult topics reflects the best of the specialty and puts forth a who's who in Oral and Maxillofacial Surgery.

I am deeply thankful to all the authors' efforts in providing quality articles that have made this issue of the *Oral and Maxillofacial Surgery Clinics of North America* a must-have in everyone's library. Last, I would like to thank Dr Dyalram for her efforts as Guest Editor. Her leadership and dedication have been key to delivering the quality that you will find in these pages.

Yours truly,

Rui P. Fernandes, MD, DMD, FACS, FRCS(Ed)
Division of Head and Neck Surgery
Departments of OMFS, Neurosurgery
Orthopedic Surgery
University of Florida College of Medicine
653-1 West 8th Street
Jacksonville, FL 32209, USA

E-mail address:
rui.fernandes@jax.ufl.edu

Oral Maxillofacial Surg Clin N Am 33 (2021) xi
https://doi.org/10.1016/j.coms.2021.05.002
1042-3699/21/© 2021 Published by Elsevier Inc.

Foreword

Management of Soft Tissue Trauma

Jose R. Fernandes, MD, DMD, FACS, FACDS
Consulting Editor

Trauma management remains one of the cornerstones of the specialty of Oral and Maxillofacial Surgery. Often, the emphasis tends to be on the management of the bony fractures, whereas the management of soft tissue injuries are often not necessarily the same situation. In this issue, we have sought to rectify this need. Dr DosSantos has brought together a group of craniomaxillofacial experts to share their impressive views on the management of this important area in craniofacial trauma.

This issue addresses the management of trauma injuries to the following subsites: scalp, nose, ear, larynx, and lip. In addition, the management of special tissues such as the mandibular unit and injuries affecting the salivary gland, has been addressed. Dr DosSantos' choice of authors to tackle these difficult topics reflects the best of the specialty and positions them well within our OMS and Maxillofacial Surgery.

I am deeply thankful to all the authors in providing quality articles that have made this issue of the Oral and Maxillofacial Surgery Clinics of North America a must-have in everyone's library. Last, I would like to thank Dr. Vatchara for her efforts as Guest Editor. Her leadership and dedication have been key to delivering the quality that you will find in these pages.

Yours truly,

Jose R. Fernandes, MD, DMD, FACS, FACDS(I)
Division of Head and Neck Surgery
Department of OMFS, Reconstructive
Orthopedic Surgery
Bayfront Health Trauma Center of Florida
1521 West Bay Street
Jacksonville, FL 32204, USA

E-mail address:
drfernandes@jax.ufl.edu

Oral Maxillofacial Surg Clin N Am 33 (2021) xi–xii
https://doi.org/10.1016/j.coms.2021.05.003
1042-3699/21/© 2021 Published by Elsevier Inc.

Management of Ear Trauma

Amir Nojoumi, DMD, Brian M. Woo, DDS, MD*

KEYWORDS

- Auricle • Hematoma • Helix • Tragus • External auditory canal • Cartilage • Perichondritis
- Avulsion

KEY POINTS

- The ear is prone to varying degrees of trauma given its position in the maxillofacial region.
- Understanding the anatomy of the ear remains paramount when repairing the ear.
- Reconstruction can take place in a staged approach to provide the best esthetic and functional outcomes.

INTRODUCTION

Facial trauma remains a common initial presentation in many emergency departments and urgent care facilities. Because of its delicate anatomy and prominent position, the ear remains a common structure that is routinely damaged. External ear injuries include simple and complex lacerations, hematoma formation, as well as varying avulsive injuries. Health care providers must also assess these patients for middle ear injuries and possible temporal bone injuries during the examination. Once an initial evaluation has been completed, treatment and repair of the injuries may proceed accordingly.

ANATOMY

The anatomy of the ear can be subdivided into 3 sections: the external ear, middle ear, and inner ear. The outer ear includes the auricle (**Fig. 1**) and the external auditory meatus, which leads into the external auditory canal (EAC), terminating at the tympanic membrane. The auricle is supported by elastic cartilage. Overlying the anterior portion of the cartilage is tightly adherent skin and connective tissue. The posterior ear consists of thicker skin that is slightly more mobile. The lobule of the outer ear consists of no cartilage. Medial to the tympanic membrane is the middle ear. This area includes the tympanic cavity and 3 bony ossicles, the malleus, incus, and stapes. The middle ear also connects to the pharynx by way of the eustachian tube. The inner ear also contains the cochlea, vestibule, and semicircular canals.

The temporal bone (**Fig. 2**) protects the middle ear and is divided into 4 distinct areas: the squamous, tympanic, mastoid, and petrous portions. The squamous portion is flat and continues toward the zygomatic process of the temporal bone. The mastoid portion contains the mastoid process and comprises the posterior aspect of the temporal bone. Medial to the mastoid process and lateral to the styloid process is the stylomastoid foramen, from which the facial nerve (cranial nerve [CN] VII) exits. The tympanic portion, inferior to the squamous region, houses the external auditory meatus. The petrous portion of the temporal bone lies on the interior of the temporal bone and encases the contents of the middle and inner ear. In addition, the petrous portion of the temporal bone is the densest bone in the human body. The internal acoustic canal is located within the petrous portion of the temporal bone and houses the facial nerve, vestibular cochlear nerve, and labyrinthine artery.

The external ear receives its blood supply from branches of the external carotid artery. These branches include the posterior auricular, superficial temporal, occipital, and maxillary (the deep auricular branch, which supplies the deep aspect of the EAC and tympanic membrane) arteries. Several nerves contribute to the innervation of the ear (**Fig. 3**). The skin of the auricle is supplied

Department of Oral and Maxillofacial Surgery, University of California San Francisco – Fresno, Community Regional Medical Center, 215 North Fresno Street, Ste. 490, Fresno, CA 93701, USA
* Corresponding author.
E-mail address: bwoo@communitymedical.org

Oral Maxillofacial Surg Clin N Am 33 (2021) 305–315
https://doi.org/10.1016/j.coms.2021.04.001
1042-3699/21/© 2021 Elsevier Inc. All rights reserved.

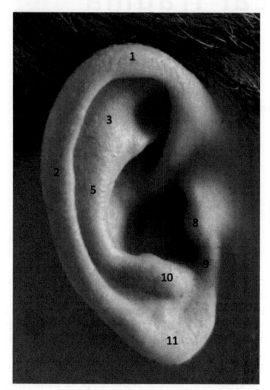

Fig. 1. Auricle of right ear: 1, helix; 2, tubercle of auricle; 3, crura of antihelix; 4, triangular fossa; 5, antihelix; 6, conchal bowl; 7, external acoustic meatus; 8, tragus; 9, intertragal notch; 10, antitragus; 11, lobule of ear.

by the greater and lesser occipital nerves (branches of the cervical plexus), the auriculotemporal nerve (branch of the trigeminal nerve), and branches of the vagus (CN X) and facial nerves for the deeper aspects of the auricle and external auditory meatus. Branches of the glossopharyngeal nerve (CN IX) may also contribute to innervation of the auricle or skin overlying the mastoid process.

SOFT TISSUE INJURIES OF THE EAR

The Advanced Trauma Life Support protocol should be followed for all patients with trauma, beginning with the primary survey and resuscitation. After initial stabilization of the patient's injuries, if indicated, a comprehensive maxillofacial examination can proceed as part of the secondary survey. If there is a noted otologic injury, it should not be addressed until a thorough clinical and radiographic evaluation is completed. Common trauma to the external ear includes abrasions, lacerations, auricular hematomas, and partial/total avulsions.

Adequate anesthesia must be obtained before attempting any repair. For small lacerations, local anesthetic infiltration can be sufficient. However, for more complex repairs, providers should consider nerve blocks. In the past there was concern for necrosis of the overlying soft tissues and cartilage if local anesthesia with epinephrine was used; however, the literature has not supported this concern and has shown that local anesthesia with epinephrine can be used in acral areas such as the ear. Studies have shown a measurable decrease in the arterial inflow immediately following administration of local anesthetics with epinephrine, but overall perfusion of the soft tissue and cartilage are not affected. The use of epinephrine-containing local anesthetics maximizes the effectiveness and duration of the anesthetic, provides hemostasis, and serves to potentially decrease total operating time.[1] Because the ear is innervated by several nerve branches, a ring block can be used to provide adequate anesthesia (**Fig. 4**). The vasculature is superficial in this area, so providers should always aspirate before injection. If the superficial temporal artery is accidently punctured, firm compression should be applied to prevent the risk of hematoma formation.

After anesthesia is obtained, care should be taken to adequately clean and irrigate the wound of any foreign bodies or debris. Simple lacerations not involving the cartilage are usually closed via primary closure (**Fig. 5**). Occasionally, irregular skin edges can be trimmed to allow better reapproximation of the wound edges. Closure can be obtained with either a fine 5-0 nonresorbable or resorbable suture. It is recommended to use resorbable sutures when repairing soft tissue injuries in children. After closure is obtained, bacitracin ointment is recommended for the first 5 days postoperatively to keep the surgical site moist and prevent eschar formation or infection.

Complex lacerations of the ear almost always involve cartilage exposure (**Fig. 6**). Motor vehicle collisions, ballistic injuries, and animal/human bites are common causes for these injuries. The ear has a robust vascular supply, as previously mentioned, and thus even the smallest areas of attached tissue should be reapproximated if feasible. Tacking sutures should be placed with caution to avoid compromising the vascular supply. These sutures can also help with surgical/anatomic orientation during reapproximation. When repairing the cartilage, figure-of-eight sutures should be placed to prevent overlapping of the cartilaginous segments.[2] Depending on the amount of edema or if any trauma is involving the EAC, a Xeroform packing or other similar material can be placed into the canal to help prevent stenosis. If there is any concern for a contaminated wound, prophylactic antibiotics can be prescribed to prevent

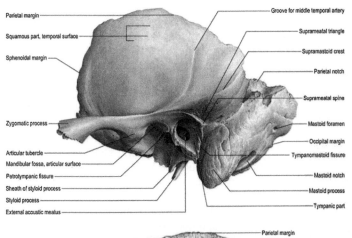

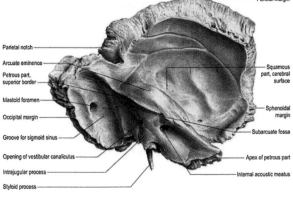

Fig. 2. Temporal bone. (*From* Waschke J, Paulsen F (eds). Sobotta Atlas of Human Anatomy. 15th ed, Elsevier, Urban & Fischer; 2015; with permission.)

perichondritis. The preferred oral antibiotic remains ciprofloxacin because it covers the main cause of perichondritis, *Pseudomonas aeruginosa*.[3] Common intravenous antibiotics include Zosyn (piperacillin and tazobactam), select carbapenems, or fourth-generation cephalosporins.

Another common injury after trauma to the external ear is the auricular hematoma. Although any form of trauma can lead to an injury of this nature, wrestlers, boxers, and mixed martial artists are most commonly susceptible. The sequela of

leaving this injury untreated is classically known as a cauliflower ear. Trauma caused by shearing forces to the pinna of the ear disrupts the perichondrium from the underlying cartilage. The perichondrium is responsible for supplying blood and nutrients to the cartilage. A hematoma then forms in the subperichondrial space. If untreated, the hematoma can lead to infection, necrosis, or loss of cartilage.[4] The resulting hematoma, if not drained, stimulates new and asymmetric cartilage to form, resulting in a cauliflower ear. Treatment success

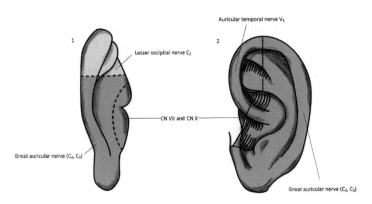

Fig. 3. Sensory innervation of the ear. (1) Medial surface of the pinna. (2) Lateral surface of the pinna CN VII and CN X.

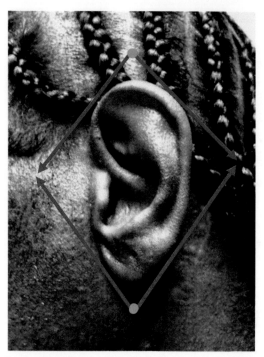

Fig. 4. Ring block anesthesia of the ear. Two points of needle entry as depicted by the green dots; at the superior aspect of the helix and inferior aspect of the ear lobe. The skin should be prepped before injection. From the superior point, the needle is advanced, traversing anterior to the tragus, aspirating along its path. Local anesthesia is administered while carefully drawing the needle back. Without removing the needle, it is then redirected posteriorly following the same principles of delivery in the anterior aspect. Next, the inferior aspect of the ring block is completed. Again, the needle should remain in the superficial plane while aspirating along its insertion path. Of note, the superficial temporal artery lies anterior to the tragus, superficial to the zygomatic process of the temporal bone. Firm pressure needs to be applied in case of accidental puncture to prevent hematoma formation.

is determined by timely and appropriate drainage of the hematoma. Methods such as needle aspiration or simple incision and drainage have both been successful. An 18-gauge needle is sufficient for drainage of a hematoma, ideally placed over the greatest area of fluctuance. If the patient presents greater than 6 to 8 hours after the hematoma has formed, the blood may have already started coagulating.[4] If no blood is able to be aspirated, the procedure should transition to an incision and drainage. An incision can be made along the hematoma, large enough to provide adequate drainage. After the hematoma is evacuated and thorough irrigation has been completed, a compressive dressing should be placed to prevent

dead space and allow reattachment of the perichondrium to the cartilage. A Xeroform bolster (**Fig. 7**), cotton rolls, magnets, and silicone dressings have all been used in clinical practice with success.[5] Quilting sutures, which pass through the external skin and the cartilage, can also serve to reattach the perichondrium. A common disadvantage is that several sutures must be placed for greatest effect. A Glasscock ear dressing can also be placed to avoid any further trauma. Repeated trauma and long-standing cauliflower ear can obstruct the EAC and interfere with hearing.[6] In addition, reconstruction of the cauliflower ear often results in poor outcomes because of the altered blood supply and exuberant fibrocartilage. Thus, urgent treatment of an auricular hematoma is always recommended.

Avulsive injuries range in their severity. Partial avulsions of the ear, even if attached by a small pedicle, should have this pedicle preserved and be repaired because a successful outcome is possible because of the vascular richness of the ear. Depending on the extent of the avulsion, the distal soft tissue edges of the pedicled segment might need to be trimmed to bleeding edges to remove avascular areas likely to necrose. The upper third of the ear is the most prone to avulsive injuries. Although any trauma can lead to avulsive injuries, animal/human bites often leave the most severe esthetic deficits. Reattachment of an intact or near-intact partial avulsion of the external ear as a free graft is often initially satisfying, but the likelihood for successful revascularization remains extremely low, especially for avulsions greater than one-third of the auricle.[7] In partial avulsions, where reattachment is not possible, primary closure should be obtained of the lacerated tissues in preparation for future reconstructive surgery (**Fig. 8**). If there is minimal cartilage exposed, careful undermining of the adjacent skin can be done to aid in full-coverage closure.

Total avulsion injuries of the ear are a time-sensitive emergency. First and foremost, if any attempt is made to reattach the avulsed ear, it must be thoroughly cleaned and free of any contaminants. Cold saline to irrigate the tissues and a well-vascularized tissue bed are vital. Any devitalized tissue or exposed cartilage should be conservatively excised. The soft tissues should be explored for any suitable vessels for microvascular repair. Depending on the mechanism of avulsion, vessels might not be available to proceed with microvascular repair. If feasible, the avulsed ear can be reattached as a composite graft. The use of hyperbaric oxygen treatment has been referenced in the postoperative care of patients undergoing a composite graft. Although there is

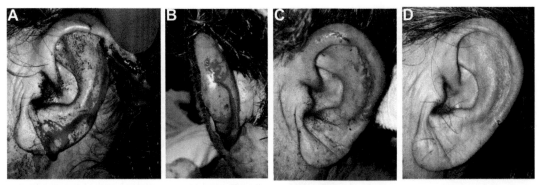

Fig. 5. Simple laceration repair. (*A*) Patient sustained full-thickness laceration from a knife attack confined to the helix of the ear. (*B*) There was no disruption of the cartilage, although it was minimally visible because of the full-thickness nature of the laceration. (*C*) The injury was irrigated and repaired with 5-0 fast-absorbing gut sutures. (*D*) Patient at his 2-week follow-up appointment.

no definitive timeline for treatment, the goal remains to stimulate angiogenesis, reduce free radical formation, and inhibit venous congestion.[8] Failure of composite grafts and other reattachment techniques can limit the options for future reconstruction. Microvascular repair of the ear can recreate the arterial blood supply to the ear, but this method is involves challenges. The first case of successful repair was documented by Pennington et al.[9] Several considerations were also noted that contributed to success of the procedure. The avulsed ear is to remain cool and the available vessels tagged. Venous grafts were used to prevent tension on the anastomoses. The anastomosis of vein grafts to the artery and concomitant vein in the avulsed ear were completed on the surgical bench, followed by arterial revascularization first.[10] Postoperative venous congestion remains a common reason for failure because finding suitable veins is challenging. Systemic anticoagulation and/or leech therapy can help avoid complications of venous congestion.[11] Another principle used for total ear avulsions is the pocket

principle. The ear undergoes dermabrasion, is reattached, and then is placed into a pocket within the posterior auricular space. The ear undergoes revascularization for approximately 3 to 4 weeks before being uncovered.[12]

CLINICAL CARE POINTS: SOFT TISSUE TRAUMA

- Comprehensive head and neck evaluation to assess for other missed injuries
- Thoroughly irrigate soft tissue trauma, prophylactic antibiotics if warranted (ie, grossly contaminated wound, animal/human bite)
- Limit excision of exposed cartilage or loose skin
- If hematoma is present, place a bolster after drainage to prevent cauliflower ear deformity

COMPLEX RECONSTRUCTION OPTIONS

Numerous options are available for reconstruction of auricular injuries. Treatment depends on

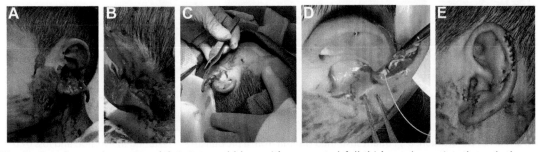

Fig. 6. Complex ear laceration. (*A*) A 6-year-old boy with macerated full-thickness laceration through the ear from dog bite. (*B*) Laceration involving helix, antihelix, cartilage. (*C*) Sutures to orient position of cartilage and soft tissues. (*D*) Reapproximation of cartilage with 5-0 Monocryl sutures in figure-of-eight fashion. (*E*) Superficial skin closure with resorbable 5-0 fast-absorbing gut sutures.

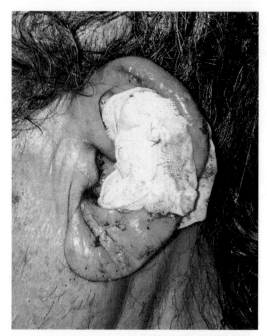

Fig. 7. Application of Xeroform bolster. Xeroform is placed on the lateral and medial aspects of the ear after trauma and secured with a monofilament, nonresorbable suture. This method serves to prevent reaccumulation of blood in the perichondrium of the ear. Bolsters stay in place for approximately 3 to 7 days after treatment.

the location of the defect and adjacent anatomy. In the upper third, full-thickness defects of the helix/antihelix, up to 2.5 cm, can be converted to a wedge defect, Burow triangle, or star defect and closed primarily (**Fig. 9**).[12,13] Significant loss in the upper third of the ear requires a new cartilaginous framework. Donor cartilage can be harvested from the conchal bowl, contralateral ear,

nasal septum, or rib. However, cartilage has no vascular supply to support a full-thickness skin graft (FTSG) or splint-thickness skin graft (STSG); therefore, if there is lack of healthy skin to cover the cartilage grafts, a temporoparietal fascia flap or other soft tissue flap must be raised to cover the cartilage grafts as part of the reconstruction. The temporal fascia is thin, richly vascular (superficial temporal artery and vein), and highly flexible.[14] An STSG or FTSG can then cover the temporoparietal fascia flap. Full-thickness skin grafts help maintain volume, height, and the complex shape of the ear to produce the most aesthetic outcome.[15] The supraclavicular areas, preauricular and postauricular areas, and inner arm serve as common donor sites. In the middle third, the posterior auricular tissues (**Fig. 10**) can be advanced and placed over the defect.[16] When considering this type of advancement, surgeons should assess the availability of the soft tissue and the patient's existing hairline. If there is suspicion for inadequate tissue quantity, tissue expanders can be placed (**Fig. 11**). Placement of tissue expanders prevents transposing part of the patient's hairline to the reconstructed part of the ear. Cartilaginous grafting might also be necessary to support the soft tissues. However, this increases treatment time because tissue expanders require a minimum of 4 to 8 weeks to achieve the level of expansion desired. In the lower third of the ear, there is no cartilage. The lobule is composed of soft tissue and has the ability to be manipulated more than other parts of the ear. Lobule defects up to 50% can be closed primarily with little esthetic compromise.[17]

Pedicle and bipedicle flaps are also options for ear reconstruction. The middle postauricular region is thinner and not likely to be hair bearing,

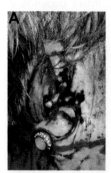 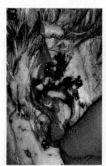 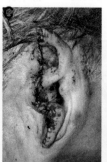 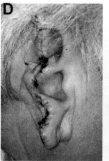 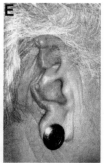

Fig. 8. Partial ear avulsion. (*A*) Patient sustained trauma from a pit-bull attack resulting in avulsion and loss of the posterior half of the external ear. (*B*) Remaining soft tissues were without evidence of maceration or necrosis. Exposed cartilage near the EAC. (*C*) Given the extent of the trauma, the decision was made to close the skin edges primarily with plan for delayed reconstruction. (*D*) Patient at a 1-week follow-up. Minimal eschar to wound. (*E*) Patient at her 1-month follow-up. There is no exposed cartilage or evidence of nonhealing wound.

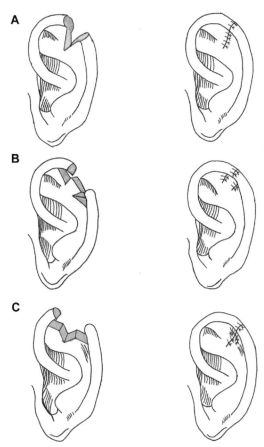

Fig. 9. Repair of helical defects. (*A*) Wedge defect and repair. (*B*) Burow triangle defect and repair. (*C*) Star defect and repair.

which allows considerable versatility in reconstruction options.[18] Pedicle rotational flaps allow appropriate coverage of surgical defects (ie, Mohs surgery) or helical reconstruction for injuries caused by trauma (**Fig. 12**). Bipedicle reconstruction, such as the tube flap, is also reliable. Here the

postauricular tissue is raised to the subcutaneous layers, folded inward, and transposed to the defect. Postoperatively, it remains pedicled to its base to maintain perfusion. After maturation in 3 weeks, the flap is severed from its superior pedicle and inset into the native ear, and a few weeks later the inferior pedicle is severed and inset.[19] Although both preauricular and postauricular tissue can be harvested, less morbidity is seen with the use of postauricular tissue.

However, circumstances sometimes prevent any primary or secondary reconstruction of the ear. Failure of a composite ear reattachment or microvascular repair leaves the patient without a viable ear. Similarly, congenital conditions such as microtia or hemifacial microsomia also result in a poorly developed or absent ear. Auricular prosthetics (**Fig. 13**) provide an option for the patient to regain a symmetrically esthetic appearance. Synthetic materials can be used to create a replica mold of the unaffected contralateral ear.[20] The prosthesis can then be anchored to titanium bone implants placed in the temporal bone. Bone-anchored hearing aids can be integrated into the prosthetic as well.[21] This method eliminates the need for additional cartilage grafting and lessens the risk of infection, graft failure, or other possible surgical morbidity.

INJURIES TO ADJACENT STRUCTURES/ ANATOMY

Supporting structures of the ear are also susceptible to trauma. Tympanic membrane rupture is a perforation in the membrane separating the middle and external ear. The use of cotton tip applicators (Q-tips) has been the leading cause of these injuries. Water trauma, assault, and acute otitis media are also causes of tympanic membrane rupture.[22] Management of these injuries is usually supportive and, in some cases, short-

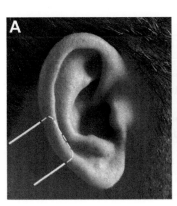
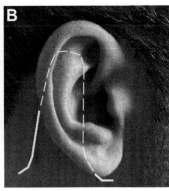

Fig. 10. Postauricular tissue advancement. The postauricular soft issue can provide many formulations for coverage of auricular defects. (*A*, *B*) Common examples of how a postauricular pedicle flap can be raised to address defects of the middle ear.

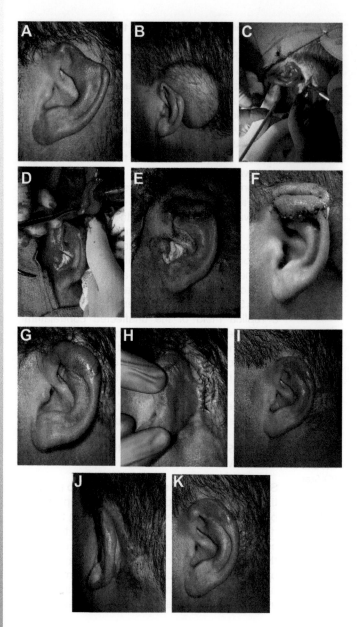

Fig. 11. Three-stage reconstruction of ear. Stage I, 0 months. Stage II, 3 months. Stage III, 4 months. (*A*) Patient with full-thickness avulsion of tissue after motor vehicle collision. (*B*) Tissue expander placed postauricular to defect to allow for adequate soft tissue. (*C*) Tissue expander removed. (*D*) Soft tissue flap raised superiorly and rotated to superior aspect of helix. (*E*) Flap adapted to superior helix and folded on itself to recreate the anterior and posterior surfaces. (*F*) Five days postoperatively. No evidence of wound breakdown or necrosis. (*G*) Local tissue rearrangement of the flap. (*H*) Closure of the posterior ear and retroauricular tissues. (*I*) Profile view at 10 days after surgery. (*J*) Posterior view at 10 days after surgery. (*K*) Profile view 4 months after final reconstructive surgery.

term otic suspension antibiotics drops can be prescribed. If the perforation is large, early surgical repair might be indicated.[23] Blunt head trauma also causes most temporal bone fractures. Intracranial hemorrhage, facial nerve weakness or paralysis, cerebrospinal fluid (CSF) otorrhea, hearing loss, and vertigo are recognized symptoms depending on the severity and pattern of the fracture. If there is any form of facial nerve function, surgical intervention is rarely indicated. Total paralysis has a more guarded prognosis.[24] Decompression of the facial nerve should be performed in a time frame of no more than 2 weeks from onset of injury to ensure the best chance of recovery.[25] CSF otorrhea is another complication of temporal bone fractures. Most CSF leaks close spontaneously within a week. Nonsurgical recommendations include head of bed elevation and neutral body positioning. Antibiotics should be prescribed to prevent meningitis. Persistent leaks may require surgical intervention,[24] which can be done via lumbar drain placement or an endoscopic transmastoid approach.[26]

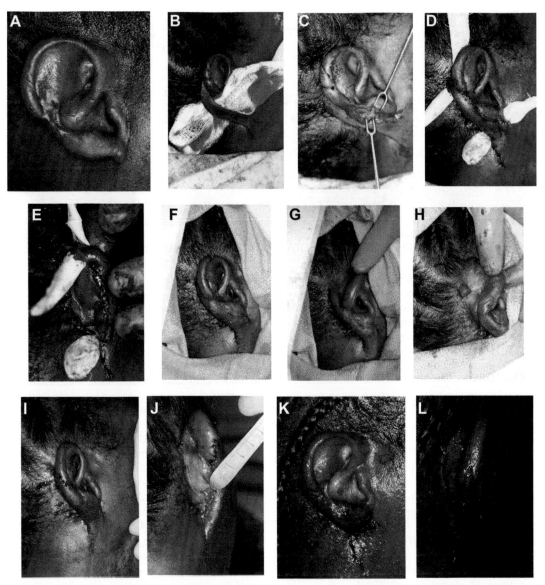

Fig. 12. Reconstruction of right ear with bipedicle flap after human bite. (*A*) Scarring and defect of the lower half of the helix. (*B*) Harvest of retroauricular soft tissue to reconstruct the helical defect. (*C*) Full-thickness dissection of the remaining helix. (*D*) Placement of Xeroform dressing to prevent adhering of the bipedicle flap to the post-auricular soft tissue. (*E*) Posterior view of bipedicle flap. (*F*) Takedown of superior portion of bipedicle flap 5 weeks after initial surgery. (*G*) Appropriate shape and perfusion of the reconstructed helix with inset of superior portion of bipedicle flap. (*H*) Excision of the stump of the superior portion of the bipedicle flap from the post-auricular space and inset of the superior portion of the bipedicle flap into the native helix. (*I, J*) Closure and reconstruction using the superior portion of the bipedicle flap from the lateral and posterior view. (*K, L*) The inferior portion of the bipedicle flap has been divided and inset and contoured to reform the ear lobule. Patient at 10 days after this procedure.

CLINICAL CARE POINTS: EVALUATION OF TEMPORAL BONE FRACTURE

- Paralysis of the facial muscles caused by facial nerve injury
- Hearing loss
- Dizziness/loss of balance

- Drainage of CSF

Many challenges exist when evaluating and treating ear trauma. Treating providers should always remember to take a thorough history, note preexisting conditions, and evaluate all clinical and radiographic information present. If there are any

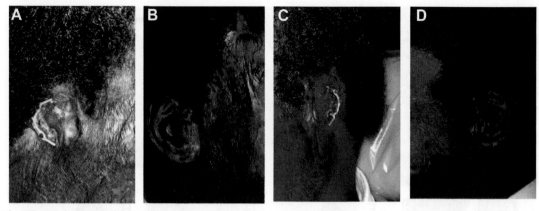

Fig. 13. Total ear prosthetic. Bilateral ear prosthetic reconstruction because of extensive facial burns. (*A*) Right ear implants with custom bar to support prosthesis. (*B*) Right ear prosthetic. (*C*) Left ear implants with custom bar to support prosthesis. (*D*) Left ear prosthetic. (*Courtesy of* Aristides Tsikoudakis, DMD, Fresno, CA.)

findings that warrant higher-level care, the appropriate consulting team should be promptly notified. Any delays can drastically alter the available treatment options and leave the patient with semi-permanent to permanent losses.

DISCLOSURE

The authors have nothing to disclose.

REFERENCES

1. Häfner HM, Röcken M, Breuninger H. Epinephrine-supplemented local anesthetics for ear and nose surgery: clinical use without complications in more than 10,000 surgical procedures. J Dtsch Dermatol Ges 2005;3(3):195–9.
2. Williams CH, Sternard BT. Complex ear lacerations. In: Statpearls [Internet]. Treasure Island (FL): StatPearls Publishing; 2020. Available at: https://www.ncbi.nlm.nih.gov/books/NBK525973/.
3. Fisher CG, Kacica MA, Bennett NM. Risk factors for cartilage infections of the ear. Am J Prev Med 2005; 29(3):204–9.
4. Patel BC, Skidmore k, Hitchinson J, et al. Cauliflower ear. In: StatPearls [Internet]. Treasure Island (FL): StatPearls Publishing; 2020. Available at: https://www.ncbi.nlm.nih.gov/books/NBK470424/.
5. Haik J, Givol O, Kornhaber R, et al. Cauliflower ear - a minimally invasive treatment method in a wrestling athlete: a case report. Int Med Case Rep J 2018;11: 5–7.
6. Summers A. Managing auricular haematoma to prevent 'cauliflower ear'. Emerg Nurse 2012;20(5): 28–30.
7. Musgrave RH, Garrett WS Jr. Management of avulsion injuries of the external ear. Plast Reconstr Surg 1967;40(6):534–9.
8. Kalus R. Successful bilateral composite ear reattachment. Plast Reconstr Surg Glob Open 2014; 2(6):e174.
9. Gailey AD, Farquhar D, Clark JM, et al. Auricular avulsion injuries and reattachment techniques: a systematic review. Laryngoscope Investig Otolaryngol 2020;5(3):381–9.
10. Pennington DG, Lai MF, Pelly AD. Successful replantation of a completely avulsed ear by microvascular anastomosis. Plast Reconstr Surg 1980; 65(6):820–3.
11. Talbia M, Stussi JD, Meley M. Microsurgical replantation of a totally amputated ear without venous repair. J Reconstr Microsurg 2001;17(6):417–20.
12. Miloro M, Larry JP. Peterson's principles of oral and maxillofacial surgery. Shelton (CT): People's Medical Pub. House-USA; 2012. Print.
13. Radonich MA, Zaher M, Bisaccia E, et al. Dermatol Surg 2002;28(1):62–5.
14. Kurbonov U, Davlatov A, Janobilova S, et al. The use of temporoparietal fascia flap for surgical treatment of traumatic auricle defects. Plast Reconstr Surg Glob Open 2018;6(5):e1741.
15. Trufant JW, Marzolf S, Leach BC, et al. The utility of full-thickness skin grafts (FTSGs) for auricular reconstruction. J Am Acad Dermatol 2016;75(1):169–76.
16. Pickrell BB, Hughes CD, Maricevich RS. Partial ear defects. Semin Plast Surg 2017;31(3):134–40.
17. Cheney ML, Hadlock TA, Quatela VC. Reconstruction of the auricle. Edinburgh (Scotland): Elsevier Mosby; 2007. p. 581–624.
18. Armin BB, Ruder RO, Azizadeh B. Partial auricular reconstruction. Semin Plast Surg 2011;25(4): 249–56.
19. Ellabban MG, Maamoun MI, Elsharkawi M. The bipedicle post-auricular tube flap for reconstruction of partial ear defects. Br J Plast Surg 2003;56(6):593–8.
20. Guttal SS, Shanbhag S, Kulkarni SS. Rehabilitation of a missing ear with an implant retained auricular

prosthesis. J Indian Prosthodont Soc 2015;15(1):70–5.

21. Mevio E, Facca L, Mullace M, et al. Osseointegrated implants in patients with auricular defects: a case series study. Acta Otorhinolaryngol Ital 2015;35(3):186–90.

22. Carniol ET, Bresler A, Shaigany K, et al. Traumatic tympanic membrane perforations diagnosed in emergency departments. JAMA Otolaryngol Head Neck Surg 2018;144(2):136–9.

23. Jellinge ME, Kristensen S, Larsen K. Spontaneous closure of traumatic tympanic membrane perforations: observational study. J Laryngol Otol 2015;129(10):950–4.

24. Brodie HA, Thompson TC. Management of complications from 820 temporal bone fractures. Am J Otol 1997;18(2):188–97.

25. Hato N, Nota J, Hakuba N, et al. Facial nerve decompression surgery in patients with temporal bone trauma: analysis of 66 cases. J Trauma 2011;71(6):1789–93.

26. Lobo BC, Baumanis MM, Nelson RF, et al. Surgical repair of spontaneous cerebrospinal fluid (CSF) leaks: a systematic review. Laryngoscope Investig Otolaryngol 2017;2(5):215–24.

Eyelid and Periorbital Soft Tissue Trauma

Audrey C. Ko, MD[a], Kellie R. Satterfield, MD[a], Bobby S. Korn, MD, PhD[a,b],
Don O. Kikkawa, MD[a,b],*

KEYWORDS

- Ocular trauma • Periocular trauma • Facial trauma • Eyelid laceration • Canalicular laceration
- Facial degloving • Foreign bodies

KEY POINTS

- In periocular soft tissue injuries, the globe must be assessed for the possibility of rupture and conditions that are contraindications to periocular manipulation.
- Lacerations of the canaliculus must be repaired and stented to prevent tearing after injury.
- Lacerations of the eyelid margin must be repaired in a multilayered fashion to prevent eyelid malpositions and cosmetic defects after injury.

INTRODUCTION

Soft tissue trauma to the face is a common injury and comprises roughly 10% of all emergency room visits.[1–3] Because of the potential for post-traumatic functional and cosmetic sequelae, reconstructive expertise is required in the repair of any facial soft tissue injury, especially to the eyelids and periorbital soft tissues. Injuries to the periocular region are often complex and involve multiple anatomic structures. Soft tissue repair with optimal aesthetic and functional outcome can be achieved through meticulous planning and knowledge of facial reconstructive techniques. This article highlights key steps in patient evaluation and management of various types of injuries, and provides a review of current literature involving facial soft tissue trauma.

PATIENT ASSESSMENT

After stabilization of the patient, a detailed history of the mechanism of trauma and patient presentation is obtained. A full survey of the face and scalp is then performed, paying attention to signs of surface or penetrating wounds, foreign bodies, and avulsed or missing tissue. Often these wounds are difficult to visualize due to obscuration by debris and dried or coagulated blood, especially in areas that contain hair, such as the scalp and eyebrows. If present, cleaning the affected areas is indicated by irrigation with sterile saline and gentle debridement with gauze. If there is a marked amount of swelling, visualization can be aided by first applying ice to the affected area. If necessary, patient tolerance of the examination can also be helped by injection of lidocaine or moderate sedation in the emergency room. Photographs of the patient with multiple angles should be obtained for medical-legal documentation.

Ocular Assessment

A ruptured ocular globe is one of the few ophthalmic emergencies that warrant immediate surgery. Signs of a ruptured globe include decreased vision, focal bullous or 360° subconjunctival hemorrhage, an irregularly shaped pupil, ocular hypotony, and the presence of blood in the anterior chamber. If any of these signs are

This article originally appeared in November, 2017 issue of *Facial Plastic Surgery Clinics of North America* (Volume 25, Issue 4).
Disclosures: The authors have nothing to disclose.
[a] Division of Oculofacial Plastic and Reconstructive Surgery, UC San Diego Department of Ophthalmology, Shiley Eye Institute, 9415 Campus Point Drive, La Jolla, CA 92093, USA; [b] Division of Plastic Surgery, UC San Diego Department of Surgery, 9500 Gilman Drive, La Jolla, CA 92093, USA
* Corresponding author. 9415 Campus Point Drive, La Jolla, CA 92093.
E-mail address: dkikkawa@ucsd.edu

Oral Maxillofacial Surg Clin N Am 33 (2021) 317–328
https://doi.org/10.1016/j.coms.2021.04.004
1042-3699/21/© 2021 Elsevier Inc. All rights reserved.

noted on the initial examination, prompt ocular protection by an eye shield and evaluation by an ophthalmologist is indicated.[4,5] Further periocular manipulation, such as examination of the eyelids or surrounding periorbital tissues, should be avoided or conducted with extreme caution to avoid pressure on the ocular globe that may lead to extrusion of intraocular contents.

In cases of significant injury to periorbital soft tissue and bony structures, the potential for concurrent eye damage should be assessed. A ruptured globe is an absolute contraindication to periocular and periorbital manipulation (**Fig. 1**). Additional ocular conditions that place the globe at high risk during periocular and periorbital manipulation, and possible future permanent decrease or complete loss of vision, include the following: hyphema, dislocated intraocular lens, intraocular foreign body, and retinal detachment.

If any of these additional conditions exist, consultation should be obtained from the ophthalmology service to determine optimum time for surgical repair of other facial injuries.

Eyelid Assessment

In the initial assessment of the eyelids, any abrasions, ecchymosis, and lacerations should be noted. The presence of a traumatic ptosis can be assessed by looking for motility deficits while having the patient follow an object in upgaze and downgaze. Oftentimes swelling will limit the motility of the eyelid, and the eyelid motility will need to be reexamined at a future date.

Eyelid lacerations are categorized as partial or full-thickness lacerations. For reconstructive purposes, the eyelid is divided into anterior (skin and orbicularis muscle) and posterior (tarsus and

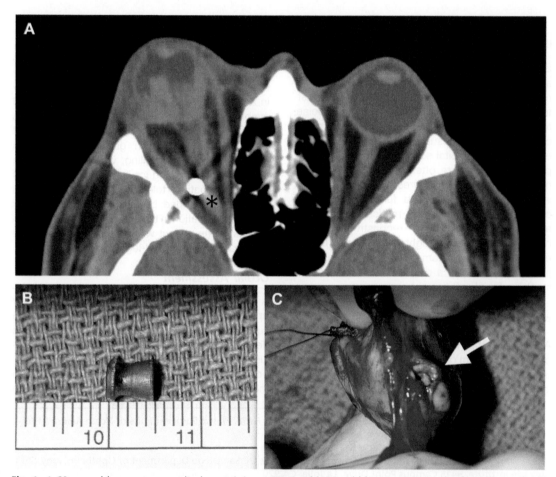

Fig. 1. A 60-year-old man was assaulted, sustaining a BB gun blast and blunt trauma to the face. The patient's vision was no light perception with a ruptured globe. The globe was found to be unsalvageable and was removed along with the pellet. This delayed treatment of his associated facial fractures. (*A*) CT-orbit demonstrating globe disruption and intraorbital foreign body (*asterisk*). (*B*) Removed pellet. (*C*) The ruptured globe and scleral exit wound (*arrow*).

conjunctiva) lamellae (**Fig. 2**). A full-thickness laceration involves the posterior lamella, and requires a more complex and layered closure. Involvement of the posterior lamella can be detected by examining the upper and lower eyelid margins for discontinuity or a notch. Some lid margin defects are difficult to appreciate on gross examination of the lid. Oftentimes an insignificant-appearing marginal discontinuity will have significant posterior extension; therefore, gentle eversion of the upper and lower eyelids is needed to assess for involvement of the tarsus. If not properly repaired at the time of injury, a large notch will be noted in the eyelid margin with separation of the eyelashes medially and laterally after it heals. This may subsequently affect blinking and the ocular surface interface. Failure to detect a marginal eyelid laceration may also result in a very noticeable aesthetic deformity that is bothersome and noticeable by patients.

The evaluation of eyelid lacerations also involves an assessment for avulsed or missing tissue. A full-thickness lid laceration frequently gives the appearance of missing tissue due to the wide gaping of the separated segments of the eyelid (**Fig. 3**). The eyelid is usually firmly opposed to the globe by the lateral canthal ligament laterally and medial canthal ligament medially; when split, the separated portions of the eyelid are widely pulled medially and laterally, mistakenly giving the appearance of missing tissue. If the eyelid tissues oppose easily with gentle reapproximation, tissue avulsion is unlikely. If marked edema of the tissues hampers this determination, gentle application of ice for 20 minutes to decrease swelling is helpful.

Involvement of the lateral or medial canthal ligaments can occur with orbital fractures or downward distraction of the eyelid. Disinsertion of the lateral canthal ligament may manifest as rounding of the lateral canthal angle. Due to its insertion at the Whitnall tubercle, rounding of the lateral canthal angle may also be seen in fracture of the lateral orbital wall. In contrast, the medial canthal ligament has 2 attachments: anteriorly to the frontal process of the maxilla, and posteriorly to the thin lacrimal bone. Telecanthus and canthal rounding also can be seen with medial canthal ligament injuries. However, further investigation through imaging is needed to assess for bony involvement (**Table 1**), as reconstructive techniques vary depending on whether the ligament is solely involved, or if there is bony involvement as well.[6]

Lacrimal Assessment

Medial eyelid injuries may involve the medial canthus and violate of the integrity of the lacrimal system. Common mechanisms of injury differ in various patient populations; in the breast-fed infant, pediatric, adult, and elderly populations, the most common mechanisms are blouse hooks, dog bite, trauma, and falls, respectively.[7–9] Medial canthal lacerations are more commonly seen in children and young adults and more frequently involve the lower canaliculus. Interestingly, upper canalicular injuries are associated with globe rupture in 20% to 25% of cases.[8,10] Therefore, if a canalicular injury is present, the index of suspicion for an injury to the globe should be heightened.

A thorough examination of the upper lacrimal drainage system is indicated with any injury

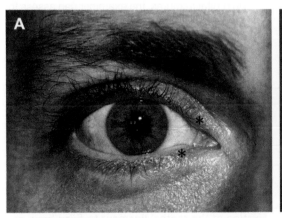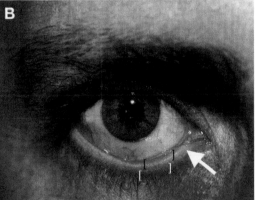

Fig. 2. Normal eyelid margins demonstrated (*A*) with black asterisks marking the locations of the upper and lower puncta. Note that the puncta are not normally visualized due to their anatomic position against the eyeball. (*B*) Everted right lower eyelid, showing the posterior lamella consisting of the conjunctiva and tarsus (*black brackets*) and anterior lamella consisting of the skin and orbicularis oculi muscle (*white brackets*). The punctum is visualized with eversion (*white arrow*).

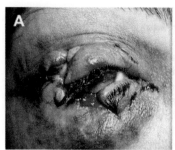 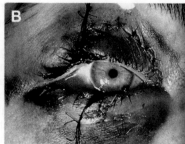 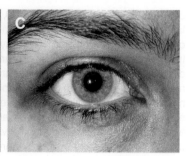

Fig. 3. A 22-year-old woman fell and hit her face on a clothing hook. (*A*) She presented with multiple full-thickness upper and lower eyelid lacerations with the suspicion of missing eyelid tissue. (*B*) Photograph of the patient immediately after repair. No tissue was noted to be missing. Note that the silk sutures were left long and secured away from the cornea to avoid mechanical abrasions. (*C*) Postoperative photograph showing a well-healed repair with minimal scarring. Note the smooth contour of the eyelid margin with absence of notching.

involving the medial canthal region or medial upper and lower eyelid.[11] Any disruption of the tear drainage system that is not repaired initially may result in chronic epiphora. Superficially, the upper and lower puncta are visible as pinpoint openings along the medial eyelid (see **Fig. 2**), and run vertically for approximately 2 mm in length. The superior and inferior lacrimal drainage system then make a 90° turn medially for approximately 8 mm, and then join to form the common canaliculus, which then connects to the nasolacrimal duct that drains through the inferior meatus into the nose. Therefore, any laceration that occurs medial to the punctum requires probing (**Fig. 4**) and irrigation to assess for the integrity of the tear drainage system. A more subtle finding may show lateralization of the punctum, which usually also suggests disruption.

Orbital Assessment

Orbital involvement can occur with deep extension of superficial wounds. The orbital septum is a fibrous sheet that serves as the anterior orbital boundary. Deep to the septum lies the true orbital fat, which overlays the 2 elevators of the upper eyelid, the levator aponeurosis and Müller muscle. Visible fat in the preseptal orbicularis area warrants further exploration, as it signifies violation into the orbital space and possible deeper injury to the orbital soft tissues and/or to the eyelid elevators. If there is suspicion for a retained foreign body, imaging can be obtained.[5] Plain radiography and computed tomography (CT) scans are the recommended first line of imaging for most foreign body materials; MRI should be avoided due to risk of metallic foreign body.[12]

The integrity of the bony walls of the orbit and orbital soft tissue contents also may be affected. A detailed discussion of the evaluation and management of orbital fractures can be found in the article by (Scott E. Bevans and Kris. S. Moe's article, "Advances in the Reconstruction of Orbital Fractures"). With regard to the periocular examination in orbital fractures, the examiner can assess for the presence of bony step-offs and subcutaneous crepitus through palpation along the orbital rim. Hypesthesia in the maxillary (V2) division of the

Table 1 Classification of nasoethmoidal fractures		
Type	**Description**	**Treatment**
I	Single-segment central fragment	Fixation of fragment to proper positioning
II	Comminuted central fragment with fractures remaining external to the medial canthal tendon insertion	Fixation of the fragment with adherence of the canthal ligament
III	Comminuted central fragment with fractures extending into bone bearing the canthal insertion	Fixation of the canthal ligament to fixed bone or periosteum

Data from Markowitz BL, Manson PN, Sargent L, et al. Management of the medial canthal tendon in nasoethmoid orbital fractures: the importance of the central fragment in classification and treatment. Plast Reconstr Surg 1991;87(5):843–53.

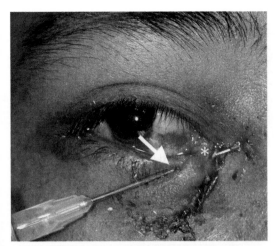

Fig. 4. Probing of the right lower canaliculus in a patient with medial canthal trauma. The white arrow denotes the entry point of probe into the punctum, and the white asterisk identifies the exit point through the lacerated canaliculus.

trigeminal nerve can occur secondary to bony impingement in orbital floor fractures, direct trauma, compression by soft tissue swelling, or irritation by localized inflammation. An assessment of the patient's vision is also required to detect optic neuropathy, which can occur in fractures of the optic canal. Last, extraocular muscle entrapment or impingement by bony fragments can be detected by observing ocular motility in upgaze, downgaze, and right and left gaze. Entrapment of extraocular muscles occurs most commonly in the pediatric population, but also can occur in the adult population. Upgaze limitation associated with inferior rectus impingement in orbital floor fractures is the most common, followed by lateral gaze restriction associated with medial rectus entrapment in medial wall fractures. Enophthalmos or muscle contusion can masquerade as muscle entrapment, and can be differentiated from true entrapment through forced ductions testing. The presence of an ocular cardiac reflex, bradycardia secondary to increased vagal tone due to tension on an extraocular muscle, is an indication for emergent release of tissue and fracture repair.

Orbital hemorrhages in the orbital space may occur independently or in association with orbital fractures. Although small hemorrhages can be observed, accumulation of a large amount of blood in the retrobulbar space may lead to orbital compartment syndrome and permanently decreased or complete loss of vision through mechanical stretching of the optic nerve or blockage of ocular perfusion (**Fig. 5**). Proptosis secondary to posterior volume expansion by a retrobulbar hemorrhage can best be appreciated with a worm's eye view. To assess for possible optic nerve compromise, the examiner may check the visual acuity and color vision if the patient is alert and oriented. The presence of a relative afferent pupillary defect is also an objective indicator of optic nerve compression and can be assessed in nonresponsive patients. It is important to differentiate a retrobulbar hemorrhage from a preseptal hematoma, as both can present as nonspecific swelling of the eye externally. However, a preseptal hematoma is not typically vision threatening, as it is anterior to the orbital septum and thus does not cause a compartment syndrome resulting in optic nerve compression (**Fig. 6**).

MANAGEMENT OF INJURIES

After stabilization of the patient, soft tissue wounds should be repaired as soon as possible. Inasmuch as most facial soft tissue wounds are not life-threatening, urgent repair of these wounds is associated with improved postoperative aesthetic outcomes.[13,14] If repair must be delayed, application of antibiotic ointment and covering the wound with sterile nonstick dressing, such as Telfa Gauze (Kendall, Mansfield, MA) or Tegaderm dressing (3M Healthcare, Neuss, Germany), is recommended. To prevent corneal ulceration and exposure keratopathy, a moisture chamber should be placed on patients with eyelid defects with exposed cornea. These can be made by placing lubricating ophthalmic ointment over the cornea and sealing the periocular area with occlusive dressing.

Medications and Vaccination Status

Previous tetanus toxoid immunization history should be obtained and administered if warranted (**Table 2**).[15] Facial wounds tend to heal well and have a low risk of infection due to the significant amount of vascular supply and anastomoses present in the face.[16] Most patients do well with postoperative application of antibiotic ointment to the sutured wounds. Broad-spectrum ophthalmic antibiotic ointment should specifically be used for periocular injuries due to risk of ocular surface irritation and chemical conjunctivitis. However, systemic antibiotics should be considered if the patient is immune-compromised, diabetic, or a chronic smoker.[17] Penetrating and animal bite injuries require antibiotics due to higher risk of wound contamination compared with other types of injuries.[17] Commonly prescribed systemic antibiotics include amoxicillin/clavulanate 875 mg PO BID for 3 to 5 days due to its broad coverage of common offending organisms, including *P*

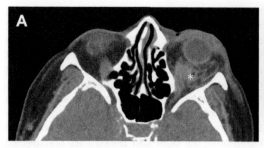
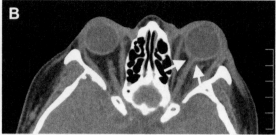

Fig. 5. A 69-year-old woman presented after a fall. (*A*) An axial CT of the orbits demonstrated a large left retro-bulbar hemorrhage (*white asterisk*). (*B*) Cross-section showing posterior globe tenting and stretching of the optic nerve (*white arrows*).

multocida (often present with dog or cat bites), however local resistance patterns and severity of injury should be considered with antibiotic administration. Additionally, patients with animal bites may need vaccination with rabies vaccine (**Table 3**).[18,19]

Irrigation and Debridement

Contaminated wounds or noncontaminated wounds more than 6 hours old should be copiously irrigated. Of note, noncontaminated wounds treated quickly have not been shown to benefit from irrigation.[20] The presence of contamination should not be a contraindication to urgent repair of tissues, as it has not been associated with an increase in complications.[21] Contaminated wounds should be irrigated with sterile saline. Surgical antiseptics are commonly used, but some reports show a possible association with delayed wound healing.[22] Debridement of devitalized tissue and

clearance of debris should be performed before closure.

Abrasions

Small wounds that do not involve exposed vital structures may heal by secondary intention. However, this is not recommended if the wound is located in an area in which a scar would cause deformation and limitation of movement of natural creases or result in cicatricial displacement of structures with scar contracture (such as the upper eyelid crease or lower eyelid, **Fig. 7**). The patient should be educated on signs of cellulitis and followed closely. Application of a nonstick dressing, such as Telfa gauze, can help decrease pain with wound changes.

Lacerations of the Periorbital Area

The use of nonabsorbable polypropylene or nylon sutures are favored in contaminated wounds, as other types of suture may act as a nidus for

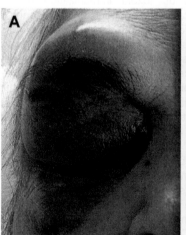
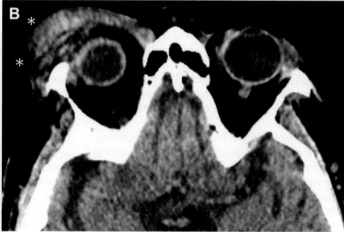

Fig. 6. An 82-year-old woman presented after a syncopal episode with loss of consciousness. (*A*) An external photograph shows significant swelling and ecchymosis. (*B*) Axial CT demonstrating a large preseptal hematoma (*white asterisks*) without intraorbital involvement.

Table 2
Tetanus prophylaxis in routine wound management

Previous Doses of Tetanus Toxoid Vaccine	Clean or Minor Wound		All Other Wounds[a]	
	Tetanus Toxoid–Containing Vaccine	Human Tetanus Immune Globulin	Tetanus Toxoid–Containing Vaccine	Human Tetanus Immune Globulin
<3 doses	Yes	No	Yes	Yes
≥3 doses	Only if last dose ≥10 y previously	No	Only if last dose ≥5 y previously	No

[a] Including but not limited to wounds contaminated with soil, feces, saliva, or other debris; puncture wounds, other wounds caused by burns, frostbite, or crush injuries.

Data from Kim DK, Bridges CB, Harriman KH. Advisory Committee on immunization practices recommended immunization schedule for adults aged 19 years or older: United States, 2016. Ann Intern Med 2016;164:184.

infection. These types of sutures also minimize inflammation that can contribute to suboptimal outcomes in wound healing, such as postinflammatory hyperpigmentation or hypertrophic scarring. However, absorbable sutures may be considered in patients who have unreliable follow-up. Tissue adhesives are an alternative option for wound closure. In one study comparing tissue adhesives with standard closure, no difference in cosmetic outcome was appreciated, and patients reported decreased pain and redness; however, the rate of dehiscence was higher with adhesive as compared with standard wound closure.[23]

Periocular injuries call for close attention to the natural skin folds and skin creases around the eyelids and eyebrows. If relaxing incisions are necessary, they should be made within or parallel to skin tension lines and skin creases. If skin creases or tension lines are not readily apparent, visualization of more subtle lines can be highlighted by gently

Table 3
Rabies postexposure prophylaxis

Vaccination History	Prophylactic Treatment	
	Total Doses	Scheduling
Previously vaccinated persons	2	Day 0, 4
Vaccine naïve persons	4[a]	Day 0, 3, 7, 14

[a] Five doses should be given in any immune-compromised persons.

Data from Rupprecht CE, Briggs D, Brown CM, et al. Use of a reduced (4-dose) vaccine schedule for postexposure prophylaxis to prevent human rabies: recommendations of the advisory committee on immunization practices. MMWR Recomm Rep 2010;59:1; and Committee on Infectious Diseases. Rabies-prevention policy update: new reduced-dose schedule. Pediatrics 2011;127:785.

moving adjacent tissue to emphasize naturally existing skin creases. Defects that run parallel to the eyelid margin should be redirected to an angle perpendicular to the eyelid margin to maximize horizontal tension and minimize vertical tension to avoid eyelid distortion. Special attention should be paid to preserve symmetry of the medial brows, as this location is less forgiving in aesthetic outcome.[24] If primary closure is not possible, small defects in the brow or forehead can be repaired with flaps based off supraorbital and supratrochlear vascular circulations.

Lacerations of the Eyelid

In lacerations without missing tissue, reconstruction of the eyelid is more involved than simple approximation of the adjacent tissues. Careful alignment of the gray line and tarsal plate is necessary to prevent lid notching and to obtain a smooth eyelid margin contour. The upper and lower eyelid is divided into an anterior and posterior lamella (see **Fig. 2**), and the 2 layers are reconstructed separately.

With large soft tissue defects, it is likely that a secondary procedure will be necessary. Hence, it is best not to use any flaps in the primary closure that could compromise future reconstruction. In patients with missing eyelid tissue, the most important variable to consider in choosing a reconstruction method is the amount of tissue laxity. In older patients, the eyelid may have sufficient laxity for primary closure despite missing tissue. A lateral canthotomy and cantholysis also may create enough laxity to allow for primary closure. If a marked amount of tissue is missing, a semicircular flap from the lateral canthal area may allow for tissue to be shifted medially to be used for reconstruction. A complete loss of an upper or lower eyelid may require a lid-sharing procedure, such as a tarsoconjunctival pedicled flap.[25,26]

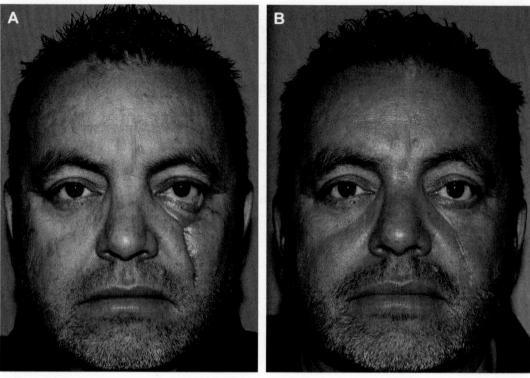

Fig. 7. A 45-year-old man developed (*A*) cicatricial ectropion and cosmetic deformity following an injury from an explosion at work. (*B*) Improvement of eyelid position after injection of 5-fluorouracil, scar revision, and cicatricial ectropion repair.

Lacerations of the Lacrimal System

A laceration of the upper and/or lower canaliculus requires prompt stenting to avoid canalicular obstruction leading to chronic epiphora. It is estimated that the lower and upper canaliculus performs 70% and 30% of the tear drainage, respectively.[27] Therefore, a nonpatent inferior canaliculus oftentimes leads to chronic epiphora and dermatitis. Monocanalicular laceration reconstructions should be considered in all cases, regardless of which canaliculus is involved.[28] Consideration should be given of repair in an operating room over a minor procedure room, as this has been shown to improve outcomes in some studies.[7,29] If there is difficulty visualizing the canaliculus for intubation, air (with the tissue submerged in fluid) or fluorescein can be injected into the opposite punctum. Viscoelastic can also be injected into the canalicular orifice to help tamponade the bleeding and identify the torn edges.[30]

There are various nasolacrimal stents that can be used in the repair of lacerations involving the lacrimal system. Common bicanalicular stents include the Ritleng (FCI Ophthalmics, Marshfield Hills, MA) and Crawford (Altomed, Boldon Colliery, UK); the most common monocanalicular stent is the Mini-Monoka (FCI Ophthalmics). Lacerations involving the upper and lower canaliculus can be stented with a bicanalicular stent, but these typically require retrieval through the nose and can be uncomfortable in a nonsedated patient. The use of 2 monocanalicular stents, or the Lacriflow bicanalicular stent (Kaneka, Osaka, Japan), may be a more comfortable option for a patient under local anesthetic only. Another option for avoiding nasal stent retrieval is the pigtail probe, which passes a stent through the canalicular system only and has the additional benefit of easy visualization of the cut end of the canaliculus. Care should be taken when using the pigtail probe, as excessive lateral traction may cause iatrogenic damage to the common canaliculus. Efficacy of stenting has not been shown to be significantly different between monocanalicular and bicanalicular stents.[29]

Secondary repair of the canaliculus is difficult; if unsuccessful, a complete bypass of the lacrimal drainage system with a Jones tube is required. Therefore, it is best to perform primary repair in the hands of a surgeon experienced in canalicular laceration repair if the lacrimal drainage system is involved.

Lateral and Medial Canthus Injuries

The medial and lateral canthal ligaments suspend and hold horizontal tension across the upper and lower eyelids. Injuries to the lateral and medical canthus are particularly bothersome to patients due to the cosmetically undesirable rounding of the involved canthus and shortening of the palpebral fissure, which is normally 28 to 30 mm.[31]

The lateral canthal ligament inserts at the Whitnall tubercle approximately 1.5 mm posterior to the lateral orbital rim and 10.6 mm inferior to the frontozygomatic suture.[32] The lateral canthal ligament then splits into a superior and inferior crus that attaches to the upper and lower eyelid, respectively. For injuries involving an isolated crus, its reinsertion to the remaining lateral canthal ligament complex is typically sufficient; however, if the entire lateral canthal complex is disinserted, reinsertion to the periosteum of the inner margin of the lateral orbital rim is required. During reinsertion, it is important to note that the normal anatomic position of insertion is posterior to the rim and 1 to 2 mm superior to the horizontal height of the medial canthus.[32] Failure to maintain this anatomic relationship can result in canthal dystopia. However, due to anatomic variations, it is best to align the canthal position with the opposite uninvolved side.

In contrast to the lateral canthal ligament, the medial canthal ligament is a more complex structure. There is an anterior and posterior tendinous portion with points of insertion at the anterior and posterior lacrimal crest, respectively. After these portions cross over the nasolacrimal sac, they fuse and divide into a superior and inferior arm that attach to the tarsal plate. Therefore, disruption to these structures also alters the normal blink dynamics and lacrimal pump mechanism, which may result in epiphora despite a patent lacrimal drainage system.

Repair of the medial canthal ligament consists of 2 parts. First, one must assess whether the anterior, posterior, or both portions of the ligament

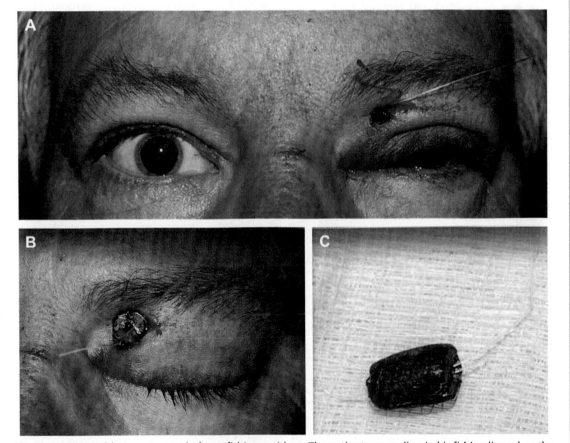

Fig. 8. A 57-year-old man presented after a fishing accident. The patient was reeling in his fishing line when the fishing weight caught and then snapped back, hitting him just inferior to his left medial brow. (A) The patient was found to have fishing line attached to a weight lodged into the left eyelid. (B) Further exploration showed a much larger and deeper foreign body. (C) The fishing weight after removal from the wound site.

are disrupted. If only the anterior portion is disrupted, an eyelid malposition is unlikely and it can be directly reattached at its original point of insertion. However, if the entire ligament is avulsed, its point of reinsertion should be at the periosteum of the posterior lacrimal crest. Second, one must assess for the integrity of the bone (see **Table 1**) and repair fractures if necessary. If no periosteum is available for fixation, a miniplate or transnasal wiring may be needed to serve as an anchoring point of insertion.

Foreign Bodies

Foreign bodies that are superficial and not located near critical structures can be removed with irrigation, sterile cotton tip applicators, or sterile forceps. Organic material, graphite, or other pigmented material (such as lead) should be removed, as retention of the material may result in permanent skin pigmentation, granulomas, infections and inflammation. Deeper metallic foreign bodies may not require removal, as they pose a lower risk of infection and removal may cause greater harm to the patient rather than no intervention.[33] As demonstrated in **Fig. 8**, it is important to fully characterize the actual size and depth of the foreign body, as deeply embedded objects may appear small superficially. If there is any question

regarding the depth or extent, radiologic studies can aid in further characterization of the foreign body.

In penetrating injuries, unwitnessed, or pediatric traumas in which the mechanism of injury is unknown, further investigation with imaging is required to assess for retained foreign body and damage to surrounding structures, particularly of vascular nature. CT scans are typically the first line of imaging for the identification of penetrating foreign bodies, characterization of their trajectory, and determining the extent of injuries. In cases of metallic foreign bodies in which imaging artifact may obstruct the surrounding tissue, plain-film radiographs in multiple views or 3-dimensional CT imaging can be used for better characterization of the anatomic location and involvement of surrounding tissues. In the scenario of high clinical suspicion but with negative imaging, surgical exploration is indicated for chronically draining wounds, persistent pain, or injury secondary to wood or other organic material.

Penetrating objects should be removed only in the controlled setting of an operating room. If preoperative angiography shows vascular involvement, intraoperative control of the vessel must be obtained before removal of the foreign body. Repeat angiography postoperatively is also recommended for reassessment of vascular flow.

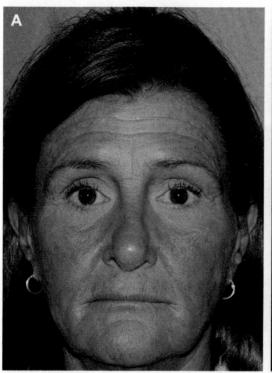
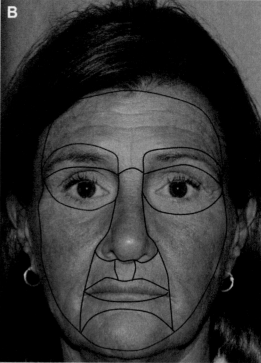

Fig. 9. Facial image of a female patient (*A*) with facial anesthetic units outlined (*B*).

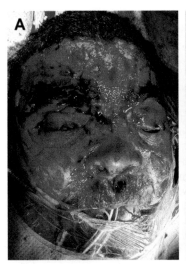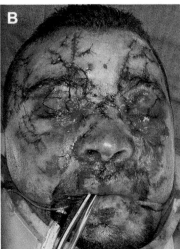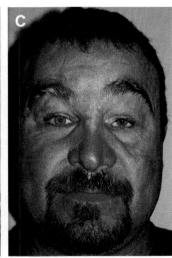

Fig. 10. A 35-year-old patient presented with multiple facial abrasions and lacerations (*A*) after being assaulted. (*B*) The patient immediately after initial reconstruction. The patient underwent numerous secondary reconstructions. (*C*) The patient at 12-year follow-up.

Degloving Injuries

Degloving injuries are a subcategory of tissue avulsion injury that involves the separation of skin and soft tissue from underlying bone and supporting structures. Vasculature is often compromised. Severe degloving injuries that involve an extensive area of skin, multiple anatomic structures, and vasculature are difficult to repair and can result in significant disfigurement and adverse functional outcomes. After an initial cleaning of the affected area with and debridement of devitalized tissues, the blood supply to each avulsed area of tissue is assessed. The integrity of larger vessels can be assessed with ultrasound; smaller vessels can be indirectly assessed by looking for areas of bleeding along the tissue flap edges.

If the degloved soft tissue flaps are viable, they are best replaced to their anatomic position. Preservation of facial aesthetic units (**Fig. 9**) can be achieved by aligning incisions, borders of flaps, and scars along preexisting creases or folds. In patients with missing tissue, it is preferable to use local advancement flaps or full-thickness skin grafts from other areas of the face (eg, upper eyelid skin, preauricular or postauricular skin) to avoid tissue discoloration and the appearance of a "stuck on" skin patch. Split-thickness skin grafts may be necessary to cover larger facial areas of deepithelialized tissue.

Due to the highly complex area of the medial canthus, medial canthal degloving injuries may present with multiple manifestations, including telecanthus, ptosis, and lacrimal involvement.[9] Severe degloving injuries may require additional

revisions after the initial repair. Injection of antimetabolites, such as 5-fluorouracil, can help prevent hypertrophic scarring and scar contraction that can result in sequelae such as cicatricial eyelid malpositions (see **Fig. 7**A).[34,35]

SUMMARY

Patients with poor aesthetic and functional outcome wear facial stigmata of their injury, and it can have a profound effect on their self-esteem, ability to retain or perform their jobs, or allow them to move on emotionally from their trauma. However, even patients with severe facial soft tissue trauma can have an excellent long-term result (**Fig. 10**). Therefore, facial, eyelid, and periorbital soft tissue trauma should be repaired with thoughtful planning and expertise.

REFERENCES

1. Hussain K, Wijetunge DB, Grubnic S, et al. A comprehensive analysis of craniofacial trauma. J Trauma 1994;36:34–47.
2. Mitchener TA, Canham-Chervak M. Oral-maxillofacial injury surveillance in the Department of Defense, 1996-2005. Am J Prev Med 2010;38(1, Suppl): S86–93.
3. Ong TK, Dudley M. Craniofacial trauma presenting at an adult accident and emergency department with an emphasis on soft tissue injuries. Injury 1999;30:357–63.
4. Chazen JL, Lantos J, Gupta A, et al. Orbital soft-tissue trauma. Neuroimaging Clin N Am 2014; 24(3):425–37.

5. Betts AM, O'Brien WT, Davies BW, et al. A systematic approach to CT evaluation of orbital trauma. Emerg Radiol 2014;21(5):511–31.

6. Markowitz BL, Manson PN, Sargent L, et al. Management of the medial canthal tendon in nasoethmoid orbital fractures: the importance of the central fragment in classification and treatment. Plast Reconstr Surg 1991;87(5):843–53.

7. Murchison AP, Bilyk JR. Pediatric canalicular lacerations: epidemiology and variables affecting repair success. J Pediatr Ophthalmol Strabismus 2014; 51(4):242–8.

8. Naik MN, Kelapure A, Rath S, et al. Management of canalicular lacerations: epidemiological aspects and experience with mini-monoka monocanalicular stent. Am J Ophthalmol 2008;145(2):375–80.

9. Kennedy RH, May J, Daily J, et al. Canalicular laceration: an 11-year epidemiologic and clinical study. Ophthal Plast Reconstr Surg 1990;6(1):46–53.

10. Fayet B, Bernard JA, Ammar J, et al. Recent wounds of the lacrimal duct. Apropos of 262 cases treated as emergencies. J Fr Ophtalmol 1988;11:627–37.

11. Priel A, Leelapatranurak K, Oh SR, et al. Medial canthal degloving injuries: the triad of telecanthus, ptosis, and lacrimal trauma. Plast Reconstr Surg 2011; 128(4):300e–5e.

12. Wikner J, Riecke B, Gröbe A, et al. Imaging of the midfacial and orbital trauma. Facial Plast Surg 2014;30(5):528–36.

13. Benzil DL, Robotti E, Dagi TF, et al. Early single-stage repair of complex craniofacial trauma. Neurosurgery 1992;30:166–71 [discussion: 171–2].

14. Aveta A, Casati P. Soft tissue injuries of the face: early aesthetic reconstruction in polytrauma patients. Ann Ital Chir 2008;79:415–7.

15. Kim DK, Bridges CB, Harriman KH. Advisory committee on immunization practices recommended immunization schedule for adults aged 19 years or older: United States, 2016. Ann Intern Med 2016; 164:184.

16. Dickinson JT, Jaquiss GW, Thompson JN. Soft tissue trauma. Otolaryngol Clin North Am 1976;9:331–60.

17. Chhabra S, Chhabra N, Gaba S. Maxillofacial injuries due to animal bites. J Maxillofac Oral Surg 2015;14(2):142–53.

18. Rupprecht CE, Briggs D, Brown CM, et al. Use of a reduced (4-dose) vaccine schedule for postexposure prophylaxis to prevent human rabies: recommendations of the advisory committee on immunization practices. MMWR Recomm Rep 2010;59:1.

19. Committee on Infectious Diseases. Rabies-prevention policy update: new reduced-dose schedule. Pediatrics 2011;127:785.

20. Hollander JE, Richman PB, Werblud M, et al. Irrigation in facial and scalp lacerations: does it alter outcome? Ann Emerg Med 1998;31:73–7.

21. Stanley RB Jr, Schwartz MS. Immediate reconstruction of contaminated central craniofacial injuries with free autogenous grafts. Laryngoscope 1989;99(10 Pt 1):1011–5.

22. Krasner D. AHCPR Clinical practice guideline number 15, treatment of pressure ulcers: a pragmatist's critique for wound care providers. Ostomy Wound Manage 1995;41(7A suppl):97S–101S.

23. Beam JW. Tissue adhesives for simple traumatic lacerations. J Athl Train 2008;43(2):2224.

24. Hidalgo DA. Discussion: finesse in forehead and brow rejuvenation: modern concepts, including endoscopic methods. Plast Reconstr Surg 2014; 134(6):1151–3.

25. Fischer T, Noever G, Langer M, et al. Experience in upper eyelid reconstruction with the Cutler-Beard technique. Ann Plast Surg 2001;47(3):338–42.

26. Hughes WL. A new method for rebuilding a lower lid: report of a case. Arch Ophthalmol 1937;17:1008–17.

27. Olver J, Cassidy L, Jutley G, et al. Ophthalmology at a glance. Chapter 28: lacrimation. West Sussex (UK): John Wiley & Sons; 2014.

28. Kalin-Hajdu E, Cadet N, Boulos PR. Controversies of the lacrimal system. Surv Ophthalmol 2016;61(3): 309–13.

29. Murchison AP, Bilyk JR. Canalicular laceration repair: an analysis of variables affecting success. Ophthal Plast Reconstr Surg 2014;30(5):410–4.

30. Örge FH, Dar SA. Canalicular laceration repair using a viscoelastic injection to locate and dilate the proximal torn edge. J AAPOS 2015;19(3):217–9.

31. Potter JK, Janis JE, Clark CP III. Blepharoplasty and browlift. Sel Readings Plast Surg 2005;10:1–35.

32. Gioia VM, Linberg JV, McCormick SA. The anatomy of the lateral canthal tendon. Arch Ophthalmol 1987; 105:529–32.

33. Halaas GW. Management of foreign bodies in the skin. Am Fam Physician 2007;76(5):683–8.

34. Monstrey S, Middelkoop E, Vranckx JJ, et al. Updated scar management practical guidelines: noninvasive and invasive measures. J Plast Reconstr Aesthet Surg 2014;67(8):1017–25.

35. Kummoona RK. Missile war injuries of the face. J Craniofac Surg 2011;22(6):2017–21.

Management of Nasal Trauma

John M. Nathan, MD, DDS[a], Kyle S. Ettinger, MD, DDS[b],*

KEYWORDS

- Nasal trauma • Nasal soft tissue reconstruction • Local flaps • Pedicle flaps • Free flaps

KEY POINTS

- Thorough inspection of the wound bed is required to account for all damaged structures.
- Preoperative photographs are important for documentation and reconstruction.
- Prophylactic antibiotics for routine nasal lacerations are not recommended.
- There are multiple options for reconstruction of nasal defects, including local flaps, skin grafts, pedicle flaps, and free flaps.

INTRODUCTION

The nose is one of the most prominent features of a person's face. Thus, repair of nasal trauma to its original form and function is paramount. Repairing the aesthetic of the nose to the pretrauma form has become just as important as repairing function. Although there may not be a functional deficit with a poor aesthetic outcome, there are potential psychological sequelae, such as depression and low self-esteem.[1,2] However, because of its multiple aesthetic and anatomic subunits, trauma management and repair can be challenging. Comprehensive management requires thorough evaluation, intimate knowledge of nasal anatomy, proper selection of repair and reconstructive techniques, and diligent postoperative wound care.

In 2011, there were more than 5 million emergency department visits caused by head and neck injuries and 41.8% of these injuries resulted in an open wound.[3] Motor vehicle accidents also account for a significant number of severe facial lacerations, with the annual incidence estimated to be more than 146,000 cases per year that require hospital evaluation and care.[4] With the high frequency of facial trauma presenting to the emergency department and other routes of presentation, surgeons need to be comfortable with overall management and the potentially complex reconstruction involved with soft tissue trauma to the nose.

ANATOMY

The nose is centered in a person's face and is one of the first features people notice. It is composed of several anatomic and aesthetic subunits that can make its repair and reconstruction a challenge. Its location at the center of the face provides it with bilateral as well as cephalic and caudal vascular supply and innervation. Structural support is critical for the function and aesthetics of the nose. **Figs. 1** and **2** show bone and cartilage components of the nose.

The boney components of the nose include:

- Nasal bones
- Frontal bone
- Frontal process of the maxilla
- Anterior nasal spine of the maxilla
- Palatine process of the maxilla
- Perpendicular plate of the ethmoid
- Vomer

Cartilaginous components of the nose include:

[a] Division of Oral & Maxillofacial Surgery, Department of Surgery, Mayo Clinic, Mail Code: ro_ma_12_03E-OS, 200 First Street Southwest, Rochester, MN 55905, USA; [b] Section of Head & Neck Oncologic and Reconstructive Surgery, Division of Oral & Maxillofacial Surgery, Department of Surgery, Mayo Clinic, Mail Code: ro_ma_12_03E-OS, 200 First Street Southwest, Rochester, MN 55905, USA
* Corresponding author.
E-mail address: ettinger.kyle@mayo.edu

Oral Maxillofacial Surg Clin N Am 33 (2021) 329–341
https://doi.org/10.1016/j.coms.2021.04.002

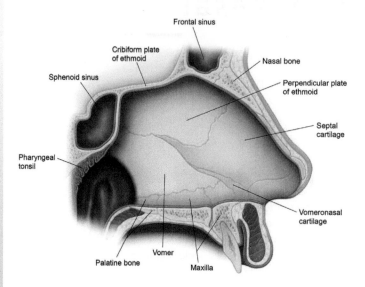

Fig. 1. Sagittal view of nose showing bone and cartilage structures.

- Septal cartilage
- Lateral process of septal nasal cartilage
- Major alar cartilage (lateral and medial crus)
- Minor alar cartilage
- Accessory nasal cartilage

External nose vascular supply:

- Inferior: columellar artery from the superficial labial artery
- Lateral: lateral nasal artery from the angular artery and infraorbital artery terminal branches

- Superior dorsum: dorsal nasal artery from the ophthalmic artery
- Dorsum: external nasal branch of anterior ethmoidal artery

Internal nose vascular supply:

- Posterior lateral: posterior lateral nasal branches from the sphenopalatine artery
- Septum: posterior septal branches from the sphenopalatine artery

Innervation.

- Superior dorsum: infratrochlear nerve from the ophthalmic branch
- Mid-dorsum: external nasal branch from the anterior ethmoidal nerve of the ophthalmic branch
- Inferior lateral dorsum: infraorbital nerve of the maxillary branch

PATIENT EVALUATION OVERVIEW

When assessing a patient for nasal trauma, a systematic approach should be taken consistently in order to have a complete accounting of the patient's injuries and to prevent missing injuries. Standard Advanced Trauma Life Support (ATLS) protocols should be initially followed and the patient should be stabilized. Once this has been accomplished, a focused head and neck trauma examination should be performed to fully assess injuries that are potentially missed on secondary and tertiary survey. Pertinent history, such as mechanism of trauma, previous trauma and surgical history to the region, time frame of injury, and functional status, should be

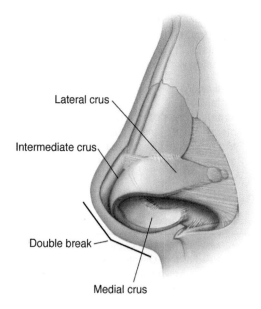

Fig. 2. Cartilaginous structures of the nose.

obtained if possible and appropriate for the setting.

When examining for nasal trauma, examination should include visual inspection of the external nose and internally with a nasal speculum examination and anterior rhinoscopy. The internal nasal passageway should be inspected for patency, active bleeding, septal hematoma, foreign bodies, septal deviation, and through-and-through injury to the external nose. External trauma to the nose should be thoroughly inspected visually and with instrumentation. Structural stability and mobility should also be evaluated with palpation. Extension into the nasal passageway, cartilage involvement, and nasolacrimal duct involvement should all be noted. In pediatric patients and high-anxiety patients, full examination and initial cleansing may have to be performed after the area has been locally anesthetized or the patient is under anesthesia. **Fig. 3** shows the importance of full irrigation and inspection in order to fully appreciate the extent of the injury. The patient had underlying fractures and intranasal mucosal involvement.

Clinical judgment should be used when obtaining imaging. Most moderate to severe soft tissue injuries warrant obtaining maxillofacial computed tomography (CT) without contrast in order to rule out underlying fractures. It is also important to

rule out other facial fractures and injuries. Plain film radiographs, including anterior-posterior, lateral, and Water views, may be obtained if CT is unavailable.

Photographic documentation should also be obtained. The damaged tissues should be thoroughly irrigated with sterile saline in order to clean out the wound and also provide representative photographs of the injuries. Thoroughly washing out the injured area allows surgeons to visualize the full extent of the injury and to determine whether there is avulsed tissue. In addition, pressure irrigation has been shown to be beneficial in reducing the bacterial load of soft tissue wounds.[5] Ideally, photographic views should include frontal, lateral, worm's-eye, and bird's-eye views. This photography helps with reconstruction in appropriate relative dimensions and potentially for future secondary reconstruction. Photography also helps with managing patient expectations throughout the reconstructive and healing process.

PRESURGICAL MANAGEMENT

A flexible reconstructive plan should be formulated after thorough examination and pertinent history is obtained. This plan includes determining timing of

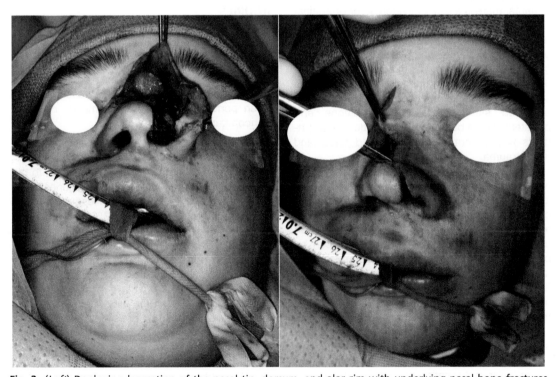

Fig. 3. (*Left*) Degloving laceration of the nasal tip, dorsum, and alar rim with underlying nasal bone fractures following an all-terrain vehicle accident. (*Right*) Wound margins grossly approximated with instruments showing minimal tissue loss.

repair, antibiotic use, anesthetic technique, and reconstruction method.

Definitive repair of soft tissue facial trauma should be delayed for emergent and urgent life-saving surgery. After the patient is stabilized, there is limited evidence for timing of repair for soft tissue trauma of the face. Many investigators encourage early cleansing, debridement, and repair of soft tissue injuries to the face in order to prevent delayed complications such as infection, dehiscence, and additional scarring.[6,7] However, there is no consensus regarding how many hours or days from initial injury is acceptable before proceeding with repair and reconstruction. Hochberg and colleagues[8] report an ideal repair time of 8 hours from injury or within 3 to 5 days if broad-spectrum antibiotics have been administered and an antibiotic ointment is applied to the wounds.

The evidence base for the use of prophylactic antibiotics in soft tissue trauma of the face is limited. Meta-analysis has shown that infection rates of soft tissue trauma range from 1.1% to 12%, with a mean of 6% in patients not treated with prophylactic antibiotics.[9] Studies have also shown that the use of prophylactic antibiotics for simple nonbite wounds has not shown a reduced rate of infection.[10] When it comes to contaminated wounds and immunocompromised patients, there is a lack of evidence for or against antibiotic use; however, antibiotics are typically given for immunocompromised patients because of the risk of severe complications. In general, clinical judgment should be used when evaluating the level of wound contamination and host factors such as diabetes, malnutrition, and immunocompromised states. Tetanus vaccinations and boosters should be updated as needed for all patients with potentially contaminated nasal and facial trauma.

The treatment plan includes determining whether the repair should be performed under local anesthesia, sedation, or needs to be completed in the operating room under general anesthesia. Most minor to moderate soft tissue trauma requiring repair in adult patients can be performed under local anesthesia. Complex lacerations, injuries with avulsed tissue requiring local flaps, grossly contaminated wounds, and complex animal bites are ideally repaired in the operating room under general anesthesia.

Thoughtful local infiltration with an anesthetic such as lidocaine with 1:100,000 epinephrine around the injury can be performed in many cases. In particular, deformation caused by the volume injected and limited use around the distal tip of the nose should be taken into consideration.

Blocking bilateral infraorbital nerves and infratrochlear nerves can be used for field anesthesia of the external nose. Obtaining true internal and external nasal field anesthesia also requires addition of bilateral transoral V2 blocks (sphenopalatine ganglion blocks) and septal infiltrations. Local anesthesia should be used for postoperative comfort even if repair is performed under general anesthesia.

The focus of this article is nasal soft tissue trauma management; however, concurrent fractures commonly present with soft tissue facial trauma. In most cases of isolated nasal fracture with concurrent overlying soft tissue trauma that does not communicate with the bone, soft tissue management, including primary closure, should be performed initially. Fracture reduction can be performed in a delayed fashion after edema has resolved, allowing more accurate bone reduction. Patients presenting with complex soft tissue nasal trauma and fractures requiring general anesthesia can have repair of both hard and soft tissues in 1 operation if it is performed before significant edema sets in. On occasion, overlying lacerations can be used to access fractures in nasoorbitalethmoid fractures. However, there is limited evidence for timing of nasal bone fractures with concurrent soft tissue injury that requires repair.

INJURIES

The prominence of the nose makes it a frequent area of damage, which commonly leads to isolated nasal trauma. However, facial trauma also regularly presents as a spectrum and combination of injuries. Thus, repair of soft tissue nasal trauma is often performed at the same time as repair of concomitant facial injuries.

Lacerations

Lacerations to the nose commonly present to the emergency department as isolated injuries or as part of polytrauma. Bolt and colleagues[11] found that nasal lacerations made up 7% of all facial lacerations. Many mechanisms of injury are seen, including sports injuries, falls, interpersonal violence, and motor vehicle accidents. Degree of severity typically correlates with mechanism of injury.

Extent and depth of the injury are important to fully assess because of possible involvement of anatomic structures in the area of the nose and adjacent to the nose. Full-thickness lacerations extending into the nasal passageway, nasolacrimal duct involvement, cartilage involvement, and artery involvement all require special considerations for repair. Ideally, simple lacerations that do not involve any of these structures are primarily closed in a layered fashion after irrigation and inspection for debris and foreign objects.

When the mucosa of the nasal cavity is involved, it should be closed as a separate layer with a short-acting resorbable suture such as 5.0 to 4.0 chromic gut. **Fig. 4** shows a laceration involving the columella and nasal mucosa that required layered closure of the nasal mucosa and nasal mucoperichondrium. Lacerations that involve nasal cartilage should also be closed in a layered fashion with the cartilage being reapproximated. This procedure is typically performed using a long-acting resorbable monofilament such as polydioxanone or equivalent suture material.[12] Cartilage edges should be closely reapproximated in order to restore the structure that cartilage provides for the nose. Nasal stenting should be considered when there is extensive cartilage involvement and concern for possible nasal passageway collapse, stenosis, or synechia formation with concomitant nasal mucosal injuries.[13] When larger vessels, such as the angular artery, are damaged, heat cautery and pressure alone may not be adequate for hemostasis. Suture tying or even vessel ligation with clips may be necessary to prevent hematoma formation. The laceration bed should be inspected for possible damage to adjacent structures such as the nasolacrimal

duct and lacrimal sac. When the duct is involved, stenting and repair of the nasolacrimal duct should be performed expeditiously because of scarring and potential complications of delaying repair of the duct.[14] This procedure can typically be done at the same time as soft tissue repair unless there are factors that warrant a delayed repair of the nasal soft tissue injury.

Abrasions and Avulsions

Abrasions and tissue avulsions of the nose are a commonly seen component of patients presenting with additional facial trauma. The level of involvement can range from superficial loss of partial-thickness epidermis to full-thickness skin avulsion and composite tissue avulsion. Abrasions commonly present with low-energy and high-energy mechanisms such as ground-level falls and motor vehicle collisions. Tissue avulsion more commonly presents after high-energy mechanisms, such as gunshot wounds, motorcycle accidents, recreational vehicle accidents, and animal bites.

Many superficial abrasions can be treated with thorough irrigation and short-term application of antimicrobial ointment or petroleum jelly to promote reepithelialization. Prolonged use of antibiotic ointment should be avoided in order to

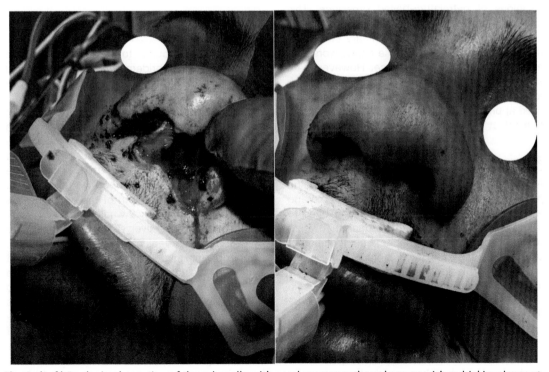

Fig. 4. (*Left*) Degloving laceration of the columella with nasal mucosa and nasal mucoperichondrial involvement. (*Right*) Primary closure of laceration with layered repair of nasal mucosa, perichondrium, dermis, and skin.

prevent delayed contact reactions and increased inflammation of the skin.[15]

For avulsed tissue of the nose, factors such as contamination level, location, thickness, and size of defect are important to assess. Pressure irrigation should be used to wash out these types of injuries. In severely contaminated wounds, multiple washouts with delayed primary closure may be necessary. However, most wounds can be immediately closed primarily after thorough washout. Location of tissue loss on the nose plays an important role in determining potential reconstructive options. Algorithms and case reviews of reconstructing soft tissue defects of the nose primarily come from Mohs surgery reconstruction.[16,17] Superior dorsal injuries may be more amenable to glabellar flaps, whereas inferior and lateral injuries may be better reconstructed by bilobed or nasolabial flaps. Thickness of the skin in the area of the loss tissue is another important factor. Distally around the tip of the nose and laterally on the ala, the skin is thicker compared with the proximal nose. Particularly at the tip of the nose, matching a skin graft's thickness with the defect thickness is important in order to prevent concavity defects. Nonvascularized skin grafts can be harvested from the preauricular or postauricular region based on the reconstructive needs. In certain circumstances, limited soft tissue avulsions of the nose can be allowed to heal secondarily with applications of petrolatum-based dressings. This method can potentially result in improved healing aesthetics versus attempting primary closure of the defect that might otherwise cause worsened anatomic distortion of the nose. However, care should be exercised when adopting such an approach, and clinical judgment must always be used appropriately when assessing the suitability of a defect for this method.

Bites

Animal bites are commonly seen in the pediatric population. In particular, children 5 years old and younger accounted for 68% of all dog bites to the face in patients less than or equal to 18 years old.[18] Dog bites can present as a combination of puncture wounds and lacerations. More severe presentations include avulsive tissue injuries. Injury to the nose and the rest of the face in toddler-sized children is thought to be caused by their similar stature to many dogs, lack of experience around dogs, and lack of understanding of canine-related behavioral cues. Standard approach to wound evaluation and repair of the soft tissue should be taken as with other soft tissue injuries to the nose and face.

All penetrating wounds created by animals or humans should be copiously irrigated with an isotonic saline solution and consideration should be given to use of a diluted povidone-iodine/saline solution because of the high bacterial load of saliva. Injuries without tissue loss should be closed primarily in a standard layered fashion. The same initial steps of wound management should be taken with injuries that have avulsed tissue. In many cases, because of a combination of tissue ischemia, necrosis, margin irregularity, and potential for infection, avulsed tissue from animal or human bites cannot be reattached. Conservative tissue debridement should be performed. Nasal reconstruction has to be performed in a delayed fashion if there is significant tissue loss that results in the inability to perform a local flap or primary closure.

Prophylactic antibiotic use in dog, cat, and human bites remains controversial. Most studies and literature reviews indicate that prophylaxis does not significantly reduce infection rates,[19,20] although Elenbaas and colleagues[21] did show that the prophylactic use of oxacillin in cat bites did significantly reduce infections. Despite the lack of randomized clinical trial-based evidence, amoxicillin-clavulanate has been the standard for animal and human bite antibiotic prophylaxis because of its in vitro broad-spectrum coverage of the most common bacteria in saliva.[20]

Burns

Management of burns to the face requires a combination of debridement, cleansing, topical antimicrobials, grafting, and definitive reconstruction.[22–24] There are many different topical ointments and skin graft materials available; however, they are not covered in detail in this article.[24] Initial management starts with identifying the depth of the burn because this guides treatment. Superficial burns that only involve the epidermis heal with supportive care alone. Burns that go to the depth of the upper dermis are expected to heal by 2 weeks with topical antimicrobials such a silver sulfadiazine, occlusive dressings, and keeping the wound bed moist. Deeper dermis involvement also requires diligent wound cleansing and maintaining a bacteria-free and moist bed. The use of xenograft, allogeneic grafts, and synthetic grafts with growth factors is common with burns at this depth.[25] Full-thickness burns should be grafted because of the severe contracture that results from the lack of regenerative properties from tissue bed loss. Wounds that do not appear to be able to undergo epithelialization within 3 weeks should also be grafted to prevent severe scarring and contracture.[25] Severe burns of the nose can be reconstructed in a delayed fashion using a combination of a forehead pedicled flap and radial forearm free flap, depending on the extent of the burn. The forehead flap provides close color, texture, and thickness match.[26] The radial forearm free flap can be used for external or internal lining reconstruction.[27,28]

RECONSTRUCTION
Primary Closure

Primary closure of nasal lacerations should be performed when possible in order to have the most favorable aesthetic outcome. As discussed previously, wound dehiscence and infection prevention start with thorough irrigation of the wound bed and removal of all foreign bodies.

True of all soft tissue closure, favorable aesthetic outcome relies heavily on layered closure that takes tension off of the superficial closure of the skin. Using long-lasting resorbable sutures such as 5-0 or 4-0 Vicryl or Monocryl for muscle and dermal layers provides the primary strength for wound closure. Sutures should be used efficiently in order to prevent oversuturing and potential for foreign body reactions. It is extremely important to precisely align dermal layers and areas such as the alar rim. This alignment helps with preventing notching when laceration involves the alar rim. Skin should be closed with simple interrupted nonresorbable suture such as nylon or polypropylene (Prolene). The size should be 5-0 or 6-0. Sutures should be removed in 5 to 7 days. Creating eversion of the wound margins helps to prevent inversion of the scar line after the wound undergoes its natural process of contraction. **Fig. 5** shows the dermal layer and skin closely aligned at the alar rim. **Fig. 6** shows the patient at 5 months postoperatively.

Delayed Primary Closure

Delayed primary closure is acceptable when primary closure has to be delayed because of emergent resuscitation and surgery. This method may also be necessary for wounds grossly contaminated with substances such as soil, oils, and chemicals. If possible, washing out the wound should be done as soon as possible and moist packing placed until primary closure can be accomplished. The same goals of strong layered closure and aligning of layers should be achieved. Conservative debridement/freshening of wound edges may be necessary if closure has to be delayed for a period of days.

Secondary Intent

Healing by secondary intent can be used in areas of the nose with small tissue defects. It is a commonly used approach in Mohs surgery defects.[29] Wounds as large as 5 cm have been reported to have been allowed to heal with secondary intent and have yielded excellent clinical outcomes.[30] Wounds in concave areas of the face tend to be the most amenable to healing by secondary intention.[31] These same principles can be applied to small soft tissue defects of the nose other than at the nasal dome. Situations where secondary intent may be advantageous include areas of tethered tissue that is not amenable to primary closure, wounds grossly contaminated with soil or oil products, and patients with severe comorbidities that make them poor surgical candidates. Advantages of allowing wounds to heal by secondary intent include lack of patient undergoing a reconstructive procedure, lack of a graft/donor site, and a typically excellent color match of reepithelialized skin. Disadvantages include increased scar tissue formation, prolonged healing time, and potential skin texture mismatch.

Skin Grafts

Full-thickness skin grafts (FTSGs) are commonly used in reconstruction of the nose after undergoing Mohs surgery. In patients with avulsed tissue of the nose, full-thickness skin grafting can be used in clean wound beds. FTSGs are commonly harvested from the preauricular and postauricular regions. These sites have excellent color, thickness, and texture match to the nose. The postauricular skin is typically thinner and matches well with the lateral nasal region, and the preauricular skin is thicker, which matches well with the dome and ala of the nose.[32,33] **Fig. 7** shows an FTSG to the ala of the nose. Postauricular skin also has less hair growth compared with larger grafts taken from the preauricular region.[32] Studies have reported fewer aesthetic deficits with FTSG compared with local tissue flaps. However, FTSG has been associated with increased postoperative infections and partial or total graft loss.[34] The use of prophylactic systemic antibiotics for FTSGs has not been shown to be beneficial.[35] Patient selection is important when deciding to perform grafting because they do require postoperative wound care and follow-up. In particular, smoking has been shown to increase partial and complete graft loss.[35] Patients also have a second surgical/donor site that they have to care for as well. Overall, FTSG can be an excellent option in

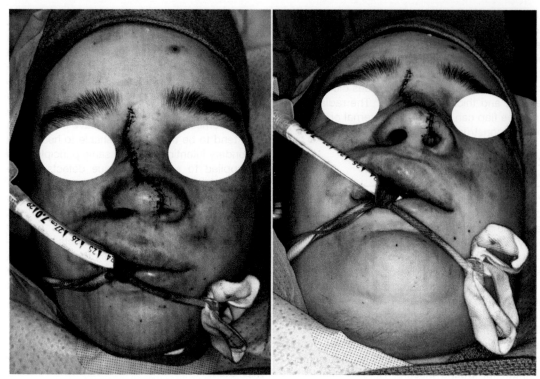

Fig. 5. (*Left*) Frontal view of primary layered closure with alar rim margins reapproximated. (*Right*) Worm's-eye view of primary layered closure.

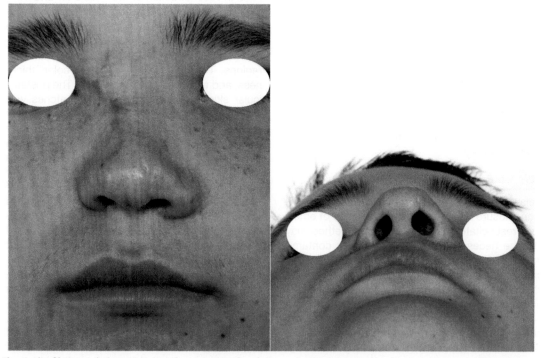

Fig. 6. (*Left*) Frontal view at 5-month postoperative follow-up. (*Right*) Worm's-eye view at 5-month postoperative follow-up.

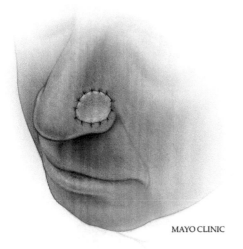

MAYO CLINIC

Full thickness graft site after surgery

Fig. 7. FTSG to the ala/alar crease of the nose.

select patients that are willing to undergo staged reconstruction.

Local Flaps

The nose has several local flap options for reconstructing small areas of avulsed tissue and composite defects. The location and size of the defect dictate which method is best suited for reconstruction.[17] The literature on reconstructing these types of defects predominately comes from reconstructing Mohs defects. Local flaps are typically used to reconstruct defects that are smaller than 1.5 cm in diameter,[36] because distortion of adjacent structures can easily occur because of the lack of laxity of the skin on the nose. In particular, the medial canthus can be inadvertently pulled inferiorly or medially. Guo and colleagues[17] formulated an algorithm for reconstructing composite defects of the nose based on the precise location of a defect. Reconstruction of the proximal dorsum and middle to distal dorsum at the midline can be performed with glabella flaps and Miter flaps respectively. Bilobed flaps have traditionally been used for ala reconstruction. For defects at the alar rim and tip of nose, the nasolabial has proved to be a versatile flap that is capable of excellent aesthetic outcomes.[37,38] Commonly used local flaps for nasal reconstruction include:

- Miter flaps
- Glabella flaps
- V-Y advancements
- Skin grafts
- Bilobed flaps
- Nasolabial flaps

Pedicle and Free Flaps

The paramedian forehead flap is the predominately used pedicle flap for reconstructing defects of the nose that are greater than 1.5 cm in diameter. **Fig. 8** shows the paramedian forehead flap used for reconstruction of a large nasal tip defect. Forehead flaps can be used in combination with cartilage grafts and other flaps depending on the defect. Patients with large nasal mucosa defects in addition to skin defects need the inner lining of the nose reconstructed.[39] This reconstruction can be accomplished by using a nasoseptal mucoperichondrial flap (if available) or, in extreme circumstances, using free tissue transfer, such as a radial forearm free flap.[39,40] Cartilage grafting can be harvested from the nasal septum, concha of the ear, or ribs, depending on amount of cartilage required for the reconstruction and availability of donor sites.

The paramedian forehead flap donor site should undergo evaluation before harvest for previous scars, previous surgeries, and distance between the hairline and eyebrow. Even small scars have the potential for compromising flap blood flow. Use of a handheld Doppler can help with more precise location of the supratrochlear artery and allow a narrower skin harvest around the pedicle during flap elevation. This method not only enables greater ease of rotation of the flap into the defect site but also minimizes the chance of inadvertent injury to the pedicle with harvest when attempting this technique.[40]

The radial forearm free flap is reserved for complex reconstructions of the nose requiring extensive outer skin and or inner lining reconstruction as well. These large tissue defects are seen with large tissue loss from severe animal bites, burns, and gunshot wounds. In addition, the forearm can be used to reconstruct multiple components of the nose with 1 flap. There are many different modifications and adjustments that can be made, including using titanium mesh, prelaminated flap contouring, and nasal lining reconstruction.[27,41,42] Complex flap design should be conceptualized and planned before surgery to ensure well-executed reconstruction. A complete palmar arch between the radial and ulnar vascular bundles should be verified preoperatively with an Allen test, and, if equivocal, should be followed with a dedicated radial artery compression ultrasonography. As previously discussed, the use of a radial forearm free flap often requires concomitant cartilage grafting and staged reconstructions

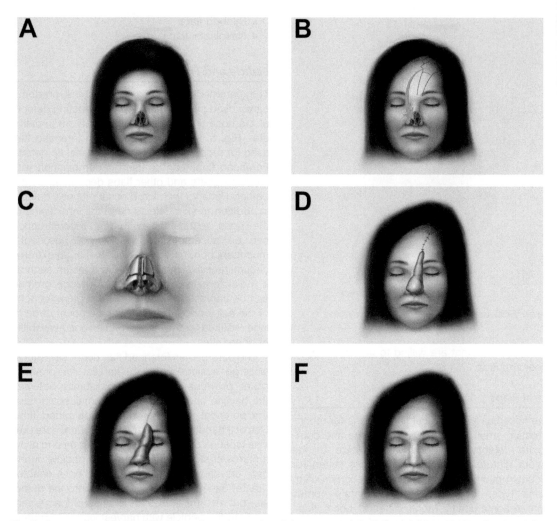

Fig. 8. Paramedian forehead flap staged reconstruction. (*A*) Large nasal tip defect. (*B*) Paramedian forehead flap design. (*C*) Cartilage grafting for structural support. (*D*) Paramedian forehead flap elevation and inset into nasal defect. (*E*) Flap ready for second-stage pedicle division after 3 weeks. (*F*) Nasal reconstruction after multiple debulking and revision procedures of paramedian forehead flap.

given the nature of nasal defects that require these types of reconstructions. When paramedian forehead flaps or radial forearm free flaps are used for nasal reconstruction, the patients typically require multiple debulking and revision procedures to attain optimal aesthetic results, and patients should be counseled on this at the initial reconstructive consultation examination.

Postoperative management

Postoperative wound care is an important component of proper wound healing; however, there is a lack of evidence-based standards of care.[43] Many types of postoperative wound care, including tape, incisional glue, gauze dressings, and occlusive dressings, have been shown to be inconclusive at preventing infections and

scar widening, and in decreasing healing time.[43] Randomized controlled studies would be optimal for standardizing facial wound care protocols, but they are largely unfeasible, particularly in facial trauma–based settings. Accordingly, the decision is generally left up to the surgeon regarding individual wound dressing preferences. As previously discussed, systemic antibiotic prophylaxis is not routinely recommended. In certain scenarios, such as animal bites, human bites, patients high risk for adverse outcomes, and severely immunocompromised patients, prophylaxis is recommended.[10,43] Prophylactic antibiotics have not been found to make a difference in patients with nasal packing for septorhinoplasty or routine closed reduction of nasal bone fractures.[44,45] However, the authors strongly recommend using systemic prophylactic antibiotics when leaving in nonresorbable nasal splints or resorbable packings for reconstructions of contaminated nasal trauma.

Revision surgeries are frequently necessary for patients with severe nasal trauma. Even if primary closure is achieved shortly after the trauma occurred, secondary scar revisions are common. A conservative approach should always be taken when debriding tissue at the index surgery because secondary revisions can be performed less invasively compared with having to reconstruct tissue that was overaggressively debrided at an initial procedure. Complications such as wound dehiscence, infection, or graft or flap loss all lead to prolonged recovery and a less desirable end result. Diligent irrigation and foreign body removal play large roles in preventing already-compromised wound beds. Although antibiotics for routine nasal trauma are not recommended, clinicians should use their clinical judgment for contaminated wounds beds. Local infection can potentially have disastrous effects. Revision septorhinoplasty should not be performed until at least 1 to 3 months after initial trauma and reconstruction.[46] Any residual functional and aesthetic concerns can typically be addressed concomitantly at this secondary procedure.

NEW DEVELOPMENTS

More recent reports have cited microvascular reattachment with survival of large composite avulsions of the nose resulting from dog bites.[47–51] The longest ischemia time for a successful replantation was reported at 13 hours because of transit to a tertiary hospital.[49] In the past, attempts to reattach avulsed segments of the nose were not routinely undertaken. However, with modern microsurgical technology, surgeons have reported reanastomosing vessels as small as 0.5 mm in diameter. In multiple reported cases of nasal replantation, a vein was not identifiable for reanastomosis and subsequent leech therapy was used. Salvage of these types of injuries is never performed under ideal circumstances and they are technically difficult reconstructions; however, the potential for better aesthetic and functional outcome remains with reimplantation versus delayed reconstruction with local flaps or free tissue transfer. In institutions that have the capability for reanastomosing vessels of the nose, consideration should be made for attempting such an undertaking when the requisite surgeon expertise and surgical armamentarium are available.

SUMMARY

Nasal trauma can present as an isolated injury or as polytrauma. Thorough examination of the nose is critical in order to not miss injuries and to form an appropriate treatment plan. Initial wound management of the nose should follow basic fundamentals of facial soft tissue management. Special considerations when evaluating nasal trauma include evaluating for cartilage involvement, nasal mucosa involvement, defects that cannot be closed primarily, and defect location. When it comes to reconstructing small defects of the nose, most of the literature comes from Mohs surgery defects. There are a wide variety of local flaps and grafts that can be used based on the location of the defect. Larger defects of the nose are difficult to reconstruct because of the multiple subunits of the nose; however, it can be accomplished through complex reconstruction using pedicle flaps and free tissue transfer. Modern microsurgical technology is allowing smaller vessels to be anastomosed and avulsed tissue that was thought to be unsalvageable to be reimplanted. Overall, wound care has seen new products become available; however, there are no standardized postoperative wound care algorithms supported by evidence-based literature.

CLINICS CARE POINTS

- Systemic prophylactic antibiotics are not recommended for routine lacerations to the nose.[10]
- High-volume irrigation should be used to wash out wounds.[5]
- Local flaps and FTSGs should be used for nasal reconstruction depending on the location of the defect.[34]

DISCLOSURE

The authors have nothing to disclose.

REFERENCES

1. Levine E, Degutis L, Pruzinsky T, et al. Quality of life and facial trauma: psychological and body image effects. Ann Plast Surg 2005;54(5):502–10.
2. Choudhury-Peters D, Dain V. Developing psychological services following facial trauma. BMJ Open Qual 2016;5(1). u210402.w4210.

3. Sethi RK, Kozin ED, Fagenholz PJ, et al. Epidemiological survey of head and neck injuries and trauma in the United States. Otolaryngol Head Neck Surg 2014;151(5):776–84.

4. Karlson TA. The incidence of hospital-treated facial injuries from vehicles. J Trauma 1982;22(4):303–10.

5. Stevenson TR, Thacker JG, Rodeheaver GT, et al. Cleansing the traumatic wound by high pressure syringe irrigation. JACEP 1976;5(1):17–21.

6. Finch DR, Dibbell DG. Immediate reconstruction of gunshot injuries to the face. J Trauma Acute Care Surg 1979;19(12):965–8.

7. Gruss JS, Antonyshyn O, Phillips JH. Early definitive bone and soft-tissue reconstruction of major gunshot wounds of the face. Plast Reconstr Surg 1991;87(3):436–50.

8. Hochberg J, Ardenghy M, Toledo S, et al. Soft tissue injuries to face and neck: early assessment and repair. World J Surg 2001;25(8):1023.

9. Cummings P, Del Beccaro MA. Antibiotics to prevent infection of simple wounds: a meta-analysis of randomized studies. Am J Emerg Med 1995;13(4):396–400.

10. Abubaker AO. Use of prophylactic antibiotics in preventing infection of traumatic injuries. Oral Maxillofac Surg Clin 2009;21(2):259–64.

11. Bolt R, Watts P. The relationship between aetiology and distribution of facial lacerations. Injury Extra 2004;35(1):6–11.

12. Lavasani L, Leventhal D, Constantinides M, et al. Management of acute soft tissue injury to the auricle. Facial Plast Surg 2010;26(06):445–50.

13. Ramachandra T, Ries WR. Management of nasal and perinasal soft tissue injuries. Facial Plast Surg 2015;31(03):194–200.

14. Drnovšek-Olup B, Beltram M. Trauma of the lacrimal drainage system: retrospective study of 32 patients. Croat Med J 2004;45(3):292–4.

15. Pratt MD, Belsito DV, DeLeo VA, et al. North American contact dermatitis group patch-test results, 2001-2002 study period. Dermatitis 2004;15(4):176–83.

16. Rohrich RJ, Griffin JR, Ansari M, et al. Nasal reconstruction—beyond aesthetic subunits: a 15-year review of 1334 cases. Plast Reconstr Surg 2004; 114(6):1405–16.

17. Guo L, Pribaz JR, Pribaz JJ. Nasal reconstruction with local flaps: a simple algorithm for management of small defects. Plast Reconstr Surg 2008;122(5): 130e–9e.

18. Chen HH, Neumeier AT, Davies BW, et al. Analysis of pediatric facial dog bites. Craniomaxillofacial Trauma and Reconstruction 2013;6(4):225–31.

19. Medeiros IM, Saconato H. Antibiotic prophylaxis for mammalian bites. Cochrane Database Syst Rev 2001;(2):CD001738.

20. Stefanopoulos P, Tarantzopoulou A. Facial bite wounds: management update. Int J Oral Maxillofac Surg 2005;34(5):464–72.

21. Elenbaas RM, McNabney WK, Robinson WA. Evaluation of prophylactic oxacillin in cat bite wounds. Ann Emerg Med 1984;13(3):155–7.

22. Engrav LH, Donelan MB. Face burns: acute care and reconstruction. Oper Tech Plast Reconstr Surg 1997;4(2):53–85.

23. Demling RH, DeSanti L. Management of partial thickness facial burns (comparison of topical antibiotics and bio-engineered skin substitutes). Burns 1999;25(3):256–61.

24. Leon-Villapalos J, Jeschke MG, Herndon DN. Topical management of facial burns. Burns 2008; 34(7):903–11.

25. Papini R. Management of burn injuries of various depths. BMJ 2004;329(7458):158–60.

26. Menick FJ. A 10-year experience in nasal reconstruction with the three-stage forehead flap. Plast Reconstr Surg 2002;109(6):1839–55.

27. Moore EJ, Strome SA, Kasperbauer JL, et al. Vascularized radial forearm free tissue transfer for lining in nasal reconstruction. Laryngoscope 2003;113(12): 2078–85.

28. Winslow CP, Cook TA, Burke A, et al. Total nasal reconstruction: utility of the free radial forearm fascial flap. Arch Facial Plast Surg 2003;5(2): 159–63.

29. Donaldson MR, Coldiron BM. Scars after second intention healing. Facial Plast Surg 2012;28(05): 497–503.

30. Goldwyn RM, Rueckert F. The value of healing by secondary intention for sizeable defects of the face. Arch Surg 1977;112(3):285–92.

31. van der Eerden PA, Lohuis PJ, Hart AA, et al. Secondary intention healing after excision of nonmelanoma skin cancer of the head and neck: statistical evaluation of prognostic values of wound characteristics and final cosmetic results. Plast Reconstr Surg 2008;122(6):1747–55.

32. Gurunluoglu R, Shafighi M, Gardetto A, et al. Composite skin grafts for basal cell carcinoma defects of the nose. Aesthetic Plast Surg 2003;27(4):286–92.

33. Jacobs MA, Christenson LJ, Weaver AL, et al. Clinical outcome of cutaneous flaps versus full-thickness skin grafts after Mohs surgery on the nose. Dermatol Surg 2010;36(1):23–30.

34. Rustemeyer J, Günther L, Bremerich A. Complications after nasal skin repair with local flaps and full-thickness skin grafts and implications of patients' contentment. Oral Maxillofac Surg 2009;13(1):15–9.

35. Kuijpers D, Smeets N, Lapière K, et al. Do systemic antibiotics increase the survival of a full thickness graft on the nose? J Eur Acad Dermatol Venereol 2006;20(10):1296–301.

36. Menick FJ. Nasal reconstruction. Plast Reconstr Surg 2010;125(4):138e–50e.

37. Uchinuma E, Matsui K, Shimakura Y, et al. Evaluation of the median forehead flap and the nasolabial flap

in nasal reconstruction. Aesthet Plast Surg 1997; 21(2):86–9.

38. Thornton JF, Weathers WM. Nasolabial flap for nasal tip reconstruction. Plast Reconstr Surg 2008;122(3): 775–81.

39. Burget GC, Walton RL. Optimal use of microvascular free flaps, cartilage grafts, and a paramedian forehead flap for aesthetic reconstruction of the nose and adjacent facial units. Plast Reconstr Surg 2007;120(5):1171–207.

40. Brodland DG. Paramedian forehead flap reconstruction for nasal defects. Dermatol Surg 2005;31: 1046–52.

41. Sinha M, Scott J, Watson S. Prelaminated free radial forearm flap for a total nasal reconstruction. J Plast Reconstr Aesthet Surg 2008;61(8):953–7.

42. Henry EL, Hart RD, Mark Taylor S, et al. Total nasal reconstruction: use of a radial forearm free flap, titanium mesh, and a paramedian forehead flap. J Otolaryngol Head Neck Surg 2010;39(6):697–702.

43. Medel N, Panchal N, Ellis E. Postoperative care of the facial laceration. Craniomaxillofacial Trauma and Reconstruction 2010;3(4):189–99.

44. Lange JL, Peeden EH, Stringer SP. Are prophylactic systemic antibiotics necessary with nasal packing? A systematic review. Am J Rhinol Allergy 2017; 31(4):240–7.

45. Jang N, Shin HW. Are postoperative prophylactic antibiotics in closed reduction of nasal bone fracture valuable?: prospective study of 30 cases. Arch Craniofac Surg 2019;20(2):89.

46. Wang W, Lee T, Kohlert S, et al. Nasal fractures: the role of primary reduction and secondary revision. Facial Plast Surg 2019;35(06):590–601.

47. Venter T, Duminy F. Microvascular replantation of avulsed tissue after a dog bite of the face. South Afr Med J 1994;84(1):37–9.

48. Cantarella G, Mazzola RF, Pagani D. The fate of an amputated nose after replantation. Am J Otolaryngol 2005;26(5):344–7.

49. Gilleard O, Smeets L, Seth R, et al. Successful delayed nose replantation following a dogbite: arterial and venous microanastomosis using interpositional vein grafts. J Plast Reconstr Aesthet Surg 2014; 67(7):992–4.

50. Macias D, Kwon DI, Walker PC, et al. Microvascular replantation of a composite facial avulsion in a 24-month-old child after dog bite. Microsurgery 2018; 38(2):218–21.

51. Akyurek M, Perry D. Microsurgical replantation of completely avulsed nasal segment. J Craniofac Surg 2019;30(1):208–10.

Management of Salivary Gland Injury

Raymond P. Shupak, DMD, MD, MBE*, Fayette C. Williams, DDS, MD, Roderick Y. Kim, DDS, MD

KEYWORDS

- Salivary gland trauma • Parotid gland trauma • Salivary duct injury • Facial trauma

KEY POINTS

- History and physical examination are integral in recognizing salivary gland trauma.
- Parenchymal injury may be managed conservatively with standard wound care measures.
- Current consensus dictates urgent repair of ductal injury.
- Cranial nerve injury should be addressed during the initial management of salivary gland trauma.

ANATOMY

Salivary gland injuries represent a small portion of soft tissue trauma but have dramatic sequelae if not diagnosed and treated. These injuries are often due to penetrating trauma but may also be iatrogenic. Salivary glands may suffer injury to either the parenchyma or the duct and range from self-limiting contusions to open lacerations. Ductal injuries may not be immediately obvious and can develop stenosis and obstruction later.

The parotid glands are relatively superficial under the skin and are therefore at risk during penetrating trauma of the face. The gland is encapsulated in fascia, which serves as an anatomic barrier that is important during repair. The facial nerve is at risk of injury, as it courses through the gland and exits anteriorly. The parotid duct also exits the gland anteriorly and pierces the buccinator muscle before entering the oral cavity in the maxillary molar region. The external carotid artery and the retromandibular vein pass along the posterior and deep aspect of the gland.

The submandibular glands rest below the inferior border of the mandible deep to the platysma muscle. The gland cups around the mylohyoid muscle anteriorly and droops over the digastric muscles inferiorly. The submandibular duct exits anteriorly and travels deep to the mylohyoid muscle before entering the oral cavity in the floor of the mouth. Nerves in close proximity to the submandibular gland include the lingual nerve, the hypoglossal nerve, and the marginal mandibular branch of the facial nerve. The facial artery enters the gland from the deep surface and exits superiorly to course over the mandible. The facial vein travels superficial to the gland.

The sublingual glands in the floor of the mouth are positioned on the lingual aspect of the mandible superior to the mylohyoid muscle. The submandibular ducts run adjacent to the sublingual glands and sometimes assist in salivary outflow from the sublingual gland. Parenchymal injury is uncommon but possible because of the superficial location under the oral mucosa.

It is critical for the oral and maxillofacial surgeon to have intimate familiarity with this anatomy, which allows prompt recognition of injury and the symptoms, aiding in the evaluation and treatment (**Fig. 1**).

PATIENT EVALUATION OVERVIEW

The authors begin their examination with A general history and physical examination. How the patient noticed the injury can be very telling, such as swelling at the area of the trauma, leaking of fluid (saliva) at the skin or from the ears, pain associated with eating, numbness of the face and lips, and a "crooked" smile or frown. Salivary gland

Division of Maxillofacial Oncology and Reconstructive Surgery, Department of Oral and Maxillofacial Surgery, John Peter Smith Health Network, 1500 South Main Street, Fort Worth, TX 76104, USA
* Corresponding author.
E-mail address: rpshupak@gmail.com

Oral Maxillofacial Surg Clin N Am 33 (2021) 343–350
https://doi.org/10.1016/j.coms.2021.04.008
1042-3699/21/© 2021 Elsevier Inc. All rights reserved.

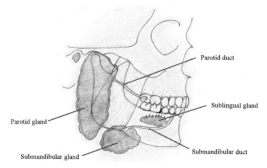

Fig. 1. Major salivary gland anatomy.

trauma itself is less critical than the injury to the structures near them, and these signs and symptoms can aid in localizing the damage. From parotid down, these adjacent structures of interest include the facial nerve, external acoustic meatus, facial vasculature, lingual nerve, hypoglossal nerve, great vessels, and pharyngolaryngeal complex. By combining the location and the signs and symptoms elicited from the patient, a focused workup can be completed. Neurosensory testing, House-Brackman scale, duct cannulation and sialography, and more can facilitate a decision of whether an injury should be investigated further in the operating room (OR) or whether it can be repaired bedside.

For a ductal injury and parenchymal injury, dye injection study with or without radiograph may be useful. Briefly, the procedure is performed after cannulation of the duct with lacrimal probe, and the duct is injected via syringe with either an anterior chamber cannula or a small angiocatheter. Dye of choice can be methylene blue, although propofol or saline also can be used and is somewhat easier to handle because of the lack of intense staining and obscuring of the field. Observation of the dye from the wound bed can be indicative of parenchymal injury or ductal injury, and if at that location the catheter or cannula becomes exposed, ductal injury is confirmed. If difficulty arises with cannulation, injection of radiographic dye and panorex could be taken to localize the area of injury.

Although radiographs are not very useful for evaluation of trauma to the salivary glands themselves, there should be a low threshold for obtaining the studies especially in regard to deep penetrating trauma. Formal sialography with contrast and then computed tomography (CT), or fluoroscopy can be useful, but requires significant coordination with radiologist, and perhaps without much more benefit than dye injection studies bedside or in the OR. As such, radiographs are more useful for evaluating collateral damage,

such as the vasculature, and CT angiogram to assess the critical vessels, such as the internal carotid, should be considered for deep penetrating injuries. A general outline of the evaluation and an algorithm for exploration are shown in **Fig. 2**, and in the next section the authors discuss the principles of repair.

SURGICAL AND NONSURGICAL TREATMENT OPTIONS
General Principles

As emphasized in the patient evaluation section, it is important to recognize the rare salivary gland trauma and damage to adjacent structures.[1–4] Ductal systems, motor and sensory nerves, as well as gland function are at risk when these organs are traumatized. It should be noted that salivary gland injury may frequently go unrecognized even with a detailed history and examination.[4,5]

Preoperative planning is vital to addressing injury of the salivary gland and associated structures. Classifying injury to gland parenchyma, the ductal system, and associated nerves aids in formulating a treatment plan. Attention should be paid to adequate cleansing of the wound and surgical exploration in a controlled environment (**Fig. 3**). The clinician should consider basic principles, such as layered closure, elimination of dead space, and suture choice. Nerve stimulators, ductal cannulation instruments, and ductal stenting materials should be available for identification and repair.

Current evidence advocates for urgent surgical repair of the injured salivary gland and associated structures.[3,5–10] Proceeding to the OR should be considered within 24 hours of injury.[7] Every attempt should be made to explore within 72 hours when associated with a facial nerve injury.[6] The ends of the transected nerve may still stimulate with electromyography during this time frame.[6] Long-term muscle relaxants should be avoided during induction and anesthetic maintenance.[9] Of course, proceeding to the OR within this time frame will need to be balanced in the setting of serious life-threatening polytrauma. Despite consensus in the literature, controversy does exist regarding conservative nonsurgical management of salivary gland injury.[4,11,12] Clinical judgment is critical when managing these injuries.

Parotid Gland Injury

Parenchymal injury
Parotid parenchymal injury is managed conservatively in accordance with general principles.[1–3,5,8] Exploration, debridement, cleansing, and closing the wound in a layered fashion are mandatory.

Salivary Gland Trauma

History and physical exam

Deep penetrating injury						Superficial injury violating the gland capsule		Superficial injury, gland capsule intact	
Acute Bleeding	Close proximity to vasculature		Close proximity to nerve		Ductal injury suspected		Clean wound and evaluate for structures within	Evaluate adjacent structures	
OR exploration vs Interventional radiology	CT angiogram		Clinical exam to confirm nerve injury		Injection study		Evaluate duct injury	Ligate small vasculature	If nerve injury suspected, follow nerve injury algorithm
If no other injury, follow general principles of soft tissue repair	Repair vessel in OR vs Interventional Radiology	If no vessel injury, evaluate other structures, clean wound and close	Repair in OR if Injured	If nerve intact, evaluate other structures, clean wound and close	Exploration and repair in OR if injury confirmed	If no fluid leak, evaluate other structures, clean wound and close	If ductal injury suspected, follow ductal injury algorithm	If no ductal injury suspected, clean wound and close	If no other injury, follow general principles of soft tissue repair

Fig. 2. General algorithm for salivary gland trauma.

Focus should be on reapproximating the parotid capsule, superficial muscular aponeurotic system, and then overlying subcutaneous tissues and skin.[3] The integrity of the duct can be verified with intraoral cannulation and retrograde injection of methylene blue or propofol. Again, care should be taken when injecting with methylene blue, as extravasation may discolor adjacent tissue and complicate repair. Some advocate stenting of the duct for a period of 2 weeks to ensure patency during the inflammatory phase of healing.[2]

Meticulous care should be taken when exploring the parotid region, as inadvertent damage to surrounding structures may occur.

Application of a pressure dressing for 48 hours after closure is useful in preventing unwanted sequelae, such as sialocele or fistula.[2,8,13] It may be necessary to aspirate fluid accumulation during postoperative visits and reapply pressure dressing to prevent these complications.[5] Some advocate for the administration of antisialagogues and avoidance of salivary stimulation (ie, nothing by

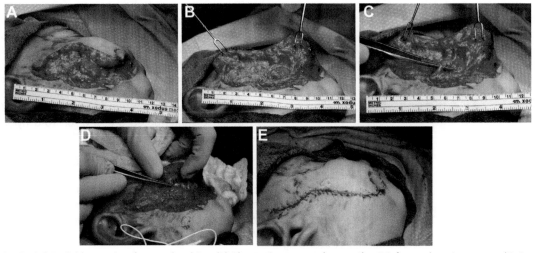

Fig. 3. (*A*) Facial laceration from a dog bite. (*B*) The patient was taken to the OR for exploration, wound irrigation, and repair. (*C*) Parotid duct identified and checked for injury. (*D*) Facial nerve branches also explored and stimulated for integrity. (*E*) Layered closure of the wound.

mouth [NPO]) during recovery.[3,5] Injection of botulinum toxin A (50–100 U) into the gland can help prevent salivary stimulation and has shown to be beneficial in salivary gland injury.[8,11]

Fortunately, isolated parenchymal injury tends to heal without significant complications.[2,3,12] A prospective study suggests that isolated parenchymal injury without damage to an intraparenchymal ducts heal 2 to 3 times faster as those with damage to the ductal system.[12] Close follow-up and exceptional wound care are required.

Ductal injury

The presence of a ductal injury presents additional challenges to management. An anatomic classification system was created to plan for the appropriate repair of the duct (**Fig. 4**).[14] Type A injury occurs within the intraparenchymal ductal system. Type B injury occurs overlying the masseter muscle. Type C injury involves injury distal to the masseter muscle.

Type A injuries may be treated with similar techniques as isolated parenchymal trauma.[2,3,5,8] Attention is focused on layered closure and postoperative management. Injuries to this region typically result in minimal complications and a quick recovery.[4,12] In contrast, it is recommended that for type B/C injury an attempt be made to identify the parotid duct and repair with microsurgical techniques.[2,3,5,8,14–16]

In some situations, either a segment of the duct is missing or damage to the duct is extensive enough to consider an interpositional vein graft.[17] Alternatively, the surgeon has the option to create

an intraoral fistula tract if the distal portion of the duct is severely damaged or unable to be identified.[2,3,5,14] The duct is brought through the buccinator muscle and sutured intraorally with a stent.[2,5]

Last, if damage precludes direct ducal repair or creation of a fistula, the proximal portion of the duct can be ligated to promote gland atrophy.[2,3,5,9,13,14] Ligation can result in temporary parotid inflammation and pain until the gland is atrophied.[3] Implementing an antisialogues regimen and botulinum toxin A injection may aid in this process.[5,11,18] Long-term studies show that gland atrophy as result of ligating the parotid duct does not cause significant facial asymmetries.[19]

The following steps describe the intraoperative identification and repair of a parotid duct injury:

1. .The patient is examined preoperatively to determine status of the facial nerve and intraoral salivary flow.
2. The patient is taken to the operating suite, and paralytic/anticholinergic agents are held. The wound is irrigated, debrided, and cleansed.
3. Intraorally, the parotid papilla is interrogated with salivary cannulation instruments or lacrimal probes. A stent (16-gauge epidural catheter,[20] lacrimal canal catheter,[8] or 20-gauge silicone catheter[1,3,9]) is then placed in the proximal portion of the duct. The stent is then observed in the wound.

Alternatively, if the distal portion of the duct is identified in the wound, a retrograde cannulation may be carried out. This can be especially useful if the operator is having difficulty cannulating intraorally.

4. The proximal end of the duct is identified by gentle massage of the parotid tissue to observe salivary flow. The proximal end of the duct is then cannulated and jointed to the distal end over the stent.
5. A direct repair under magnification (loupes or OR microscope) is made using nonresorbable suture material. Literature supports the use of at least 3 interrupted 8-0, 9-0, or 10-0 nylon sutures.[2,3,8,9,17]

Alternatively, if the distal end of the duct is unable to be identified or repaired, a fistula can be created. Hemostats are passed through the buccinator muscle and mucosa. The proximal duct is then brought through the tunnel and secured to the mucosa with 8-0 nylon.[3]

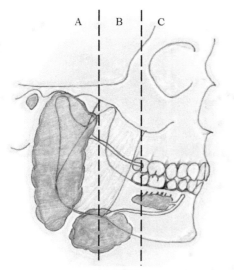

Fig. 4. Classifications of parotid duct injury according to Van Sickels.[14] *Data from* Van Sickels JE. Parotid duct injuries. *Oral Surg Oral Med Oral Pathol.* 1981;52(4):364-367.

6. The intraoral portion of the stent is then sutured in place for approximately 2 weeks.

7. Finally, the wound is closed in a layered fashion. Consideration is given to injection of botulinum toxin A, pressure dressings, use of antisialagogues as well as a period of NPO.

Facial nerve injury

Facial nerve injury should be suspected when dealing with injuries involving the parotid gland. In a prospective study, isolated glandular injury was associated with a 20% risk of facial nerve injury. Incidence increased to 55% when the parotid duct was injured.[21] The buccal branch of the facial nerve is most commonly injured, as it is closely associated with the parotid duct.[5] Preoperative assessment is often a good predictor of facial nerve function and should be documented before repair attempts.

Current recommendations support primary repair of facial nerve transection.[6,7] Nerve transection proximal to a vertical line between lateral canthus and mental foramen is a candidate for repair.[8] Excellent functional results are typically observed.[7] Again, neuromuscular relaxing agents should be avoided, and an attempt should be made to identify and repair nerve injuries within 72 hours. After this time frame, neurotransmitter stores are depleted and will not respond to nerve stimulation, thus creating difficulty in identifying proximal and distal nerve stumps.[6,8] Neurorrhaphy and grafting techniques are well described in the literature.[6,8] An additional discussion on specific nerve repair techniques can be found in a subsequent article.

Submandibular and Sublingual Gland Injury

Submandibular and sublingual gland trauma is quite rare. The body of the mandible serves as anatomic protection to both glands.[2,5,22] Mandibular body fractures, penetrating wounds, and ballistic injury (self-inflicted) can lead to submandibular and sublingual gland trauma. Intraoral trauma to Wharton duct may lead to sialadenitis of both glands. Again, it is important to assess the function of adjacent structures. The clinician should assess the marginal mandibular branch of the facial nerve (in submandibular gland trauma) and lingual nerve injury (both sublingual and submandibular gland trauma).

Isolated parenchymal injury to these glands can be managed similarly to parotid gland trauma. Irrigation, debridement, layered closure, pressure dressings, and close follow-up form the foundation of treatment. Submandibular gland trauma has been found to respond well to conservative treatment.[22] Damage to Wharton duct should be treated with marsupialization of the duct at the site of injury to prevent sialocele.[5,23]

The clinician should have a low threshold to excise the sublingual or submandibular gland if injury is significant because the morbidity is low for these procedures.[2,5,24] A concerted effort to identify nerve injury should be made. Primary repair often provides the highest chance for nerve recovery.[6]

Minor Salivary Gland Injury

There are approximately 800 to 1000 minor salivary glands within the upper aerodigestive tract.[25] Injury to minor salivary glands can occur with intraoral trauma. Treatment of intraoral wounds focuses on basic principles as discussed previously. Minor salivary glands that appear to be injured can be easily removed during primary repair. Mucocele may form from complications of minor salivary gland trauma and is treated with excising the offending and surrounding glands.[26]

Management of Complications

Salivary gland trauma presents with unique challenges for management. Complications arising from unrecognized injury and appropriate treatment can significantly alter quality of life. Luckily, many complications that arise from salivary gland trauma can be managed conservatively.[5,7,11,12,18,21,22] However, there are instances in which surgical intervention is warranted.[27–29] Complications arising for gland trauma include infection, sialocele, fistula, and auriculotemporal syndrome.

Infection

The best prevention for postoperative infection includes adherence to basic principles of soft tissue wound management. Timely repair, adequate would debridement, and cleansing with antimicrobials (polyhexanide, povidone iodine) cannot be overstated. Consideration should be given to prophylactic antibiotic therapy in especially severe trauma to the gland.[8] Coverage should be directed against *Streptococcus* spp, *Staphylococcus* spp, as well as *Haemophilus influenzae*. The duration of antibiotic coverage is 1 to 2 weeks and can be extended for the duration of stent usage.[2,3,5,8,20] Grossly infected wounds are managed with serial irrigation and debridement.

Sialocele

A sialocele is a fluid-filled cavity that has resulted from saliva extravasation. Sialocele typically develops 1 to 2 weeks after salivary gland trauma and results in soft swellings adjacent to the gland.[2,5] Diagnosis is made by physical examination combined with fluid aspirate analysis (amylase levels >10,000 U/L).[3,10]

Conservative management is favored as initial treatment and includes application of pressure dressings, repeated fluid aspiration, limited oral intake/NPO, antisialogogues, and administration of antibiotics.[1,2,5,9] Stenting of the duct may aid in the resolution of a sialocele.[13] Glandular injection of botulinum toxin A has shown promise in treating sialocele following trauma.[11,18] Fifty to 100 IU is injected with care to avoid adjacent structures. It should be noted that, although response to nonsurgical treatment of sialocele is usually timely, patience and long-term management may be required.

Recently, endoscopic techniques have demonstrated effectiveness in the management of sialocele following gland injury.[29] Success with this technique requires operator experience.[30,31] Surgical exploration and local excision of persistent sialocele have been reported.[27,28] Gland excision is the final option in sialocele management; however, this should be reserved for truly intractable cases.[2,5] Gland excision in the presence of scar tissue and contracture is technically challenging and can result in iatrogenic damage to the facial nerve.[32] Last, radiation therapy to treat complications of salivary gland injury is no longer recommended, as it can lead to malignant transformation.[2,5]

Salivary fistula

Cutaneous fistulae are tracts that communicate between gland tissue and skin and result in external drainage of saliva. Unlike sialocele, salivary fistulae are typically observed within the first week after injury.[5] Fistulae can develop after closing a wound over an unrecognized ducal injury or as the result of ruptured sialocele through skin. Physical examination as well as fluid analysis for amylase is diagnostic. Conservative management is again favored as initial treatment.

Methods used in the treatment of sialocele are applied to the treatment of fistula. Both retrospective and prospective studies have shown good response to fistula resolution with nonsurgical conservative management; however, surgical treatment may be indicated.[7,12] Again, the clinician should understand that nonsurgical management of salivary gland fistula can take a protracted course.

Auriculotemporal syndrome

Auriculotemporal syndrome (also known as Frey syndrome or gustatory sweating) is a commonly encountered sequela of parotid surgery.[33] Frey syndrome has also been reported after facial trauma.[34] The syndrome is a result of aberrant regeneration of postganglionic parasympathetic fibers innervating the skin surrounding an insult to the parotid region.[5,33] Patients who are affected complain of flushing or sweating of the overlying skin in response to salivation or mastication.[33] The syndrome can be diagnosed on history and clinical examination in conjunction with a starch iodine test. Current treatment regimens include topical application of anticholinergics or injection of botulinum toxin A.[3,9,33]

NEW DEVELOPMENTS

There are not too many new developments for evaluation of ductal injury. A search of the literature of salivary gland injury via PubMed found only 324 articles available, with many being a review article or associated with radiation injury.

There are, however, efforts to use regenerative medicine for salivary trauma. Porcheri and Mitsiadis[35] discuss a general review of regenerative options, starting with stem cell therapies. Given that general healing for salivary glands, the cells are bound to "fate-commitment program," using transcription factors, studies show promise in regenerating of all cell types of the parotid parenchyma.[36,37] However, this is still under investigation, and as with many general stem cell therapies, concerns of promoting cancer cells or conversion to cancer stem cells remain.

Three-dimensional scaffolds and bioengineering the salivary gland also have been under investigation. However, limitation of short lifespan of the salivary gland cells has hampered further development for now, although using cells of a different timeline could yield more stable organs that can live long enough for organ generation.[35] Although some of the basic science research efforts and the theory show promise, the clinical application of these methods is still in its early stages.

SUMMARY

Salivary gland trauma can result from soft tissue injury to the maxillofacial region. The first step in management includes a thorough evaluation for injury to salivary glands and associated structures. Recognizing injury to the parenchyma, ductal system, and associated neurovascular structures is imperative to executing proper treatment. Parenchymal injury is managed conservatively with cleansing, gentile debridement, layered closure, and application of pressure dressings with good results. Ductal injury should be explored and treated urgently using microsurgical techniques. Associated facial nerve injury should be treated with primary repair within 72 hours when possible. Adjuncts, such as botulinum toxin A, periods of

NPO, and antisialagogues, have been shown to be beneficial in treating injuries.

Complications may arise in treated and untreated salivary gland injury. The most common complications include infection, sialocele, and fistula. Treatment of complications can range from conservative management to excision of the offending gland. Nonsurgical management of complications may take a protracted course. Again, the use of adjuncts is useful in managing complications involving salivary gland injury. Minimally invasive techniques may also have a role in managing salivary gland injury. There is current interest in bioengineering and regenerative medicine that may impact the way salivary gland injury is managed in the future.

CLINICS CARE POINTS

- Careful history and physical examination are the most reliable method of diagnosing salivary gland injury.
- Isolated parenchymal injury may be managed conservatively with low risk for postoperative complications.
- Acute repair of ductal injuries via microsurgical techniques is suggested within 24 hours of injury.
- Concomitant cranial nerve injury should be evaluated and treated within 72 hours for best outcomes.
- Botulinum toxin A, compressive dressings, and antisialagogues are useful adjuncts in treating primary injury and secondary complications of salivary gland trauma.

DISCLOSURE

The authors have nothing to disclose.

REFERENCES

1. Flint P, Haughey B, Lund V, et al. Cummings Otolaryngology: Head and Neck Surgery. 6th edition. Philadelphia: Mosby Elsevier; 2014.
2. Lazaridou M, Iliopoulos C, Antoniades K, et al. Salivary gland trauma: a review of diagnosis and treatment. Craniomaxillofac Trauma Reconstr 2012;5(4):189–96.
3. Gordin EA, Daniero JJ, Krein H, et al. Parotid gland trauma. Facial Plast Surg 2010;26(6):504–10.
4. Lewis G, Knottenbelt JD. Parotid duct injury: is immediate surgical repair necessary? Injury 1991; 22(5):407–9.
5. Fonseca R, Barber HD, Powers M, et al. Oral and Maxillofacial Trauma. 4th edition. Saunders; 2012.
6. Greywoode JD, Ho HH, Artz GJ, et al. Management of traumatic facial nerve injuries. Facial Plast Surg 2010;26(6):511–8.
7. Tachmes L, Woloszyn T, Marini C, et al. Parotid gland and facial nerve trauma: a retrospective review. J Trauma 1990;30(11):1395–8.
8. Tisch M, Maier S, Maier H. Penetrating trauma to the parotid gland. Facial Plast Surg 2015;31(4):376–81.
9. Steinberg MJ, Herrera AF. Management of parotid duct injuries. Oral Surg Oral Med Oral Pathol Oral Radiol Endod 2005;99(2):136–41.
10. Lewkowicz AA, Hasson O, Nahlieli O. Traumatic injuries to the parotid gland and duct. J Oral Maxillofac Surg 2002;60(6):676–80.
11. Arnaud S, Batifol D, Goudot P, et al. Nonsurgical management of traumatic injuries of the parotid gland and duct using type a botulinum toxin. Plast Reconstr Surg 2006;117(7):2426–30.
12. Parekh D, Glezerson G, Stewart M, et al. Post-traumatic parotid fistulae and sialoceles. A prospective study of conservative management in 51 cases. Ann Surg 1989;209(1):105–11.
13. Epker BN, Burnette JC. Trauma to the parotid gland and duct: primary treatment and management of complications. J Oral Surg 1970;28(9):657–70.
14. Van Sickels JE. Parotid duct injuries. Oral Surg Oral Med Oral Pathol 1981;52(4):364–7.
15. Hallock GG. Microsurgical repair of the parotid duct. Microsurgery 1992;13(5):243–6.
16. Youngs RP, Walsh-Waring GP. Trauma to the parotid region. J Laryngol Otol 1987;101(5):475–9.
17. Heymans O, Nélissen X, Médot M, et al. Microsurgical repair of Stensen's duct using an interposition vein graft. J Reconstr Microsurg 1999;15(2):105–8.
18. Costan V-V, Dabija MG, Ciofu ML, et al. A functional approach to posttraumatic salivary fistula treatment: the use of botulinum toxin. J Craniofac Surg 2019; 30(3):871–5.
19. Baron HC. Parotid gland atrophy. Arch Surg 1962; 85(6):1042.
20. Sujeeth S, Dindawar S. Parotid duct repair using an epidural catheter. Int J Oral Maxillofac Surg 2011; 40(7):747–8.
21. Landau R, Stewart M. Conservative management of post-traumatic parotid fistulae and sialoceles: a prospective study. Br J Surg 1985;72(1):42–4.
22. Singh B, Shaha A. Traumatic submandibular salivary gland fistula. J Oral Maxillofac Surg 1995;53(3): 338–9.
23. Baurmash HD. Marsupialization for treatment of oral ranula: a second look at the procedure. J Oral Maxillofac Surg 1992;50(12):1274–9.
24. Nadershah M, Salama A. Removal of parotid, submandibular, and sublingual glands. Oral Maxillofac Surg Clin North Am 2012;24(2):295–305, x.

25. Kessler AT, Bhatt AA. Review of the major and minor salivary glands, part 1: anatomy, infectious, and inflammatory processes. J Clin Imaging Sci 2018;8:47.

26. Yamasoba T, Tayama N, Syoji M, et al. Clinicostatistical study of lower lip mucoceles. Head Neck 1990; 12(4):316–20.

27. Kulkarni A, Chandrasala S, Nimbeni BS, et al. Management of an unusual case of iatrogenic parotid sialocele using an infant feeding tube: a novel approach. BMJ Case Rep 2014;2014. bcr2014205845.

28. Hwang J, You YC, Burm JS. Treatment of intractable parotid sialocele occurred after open reduction-fixation of mandibular subcondylar fracture. Arch Craniofac Surg 2018;19(2):157–61.

29. Nahlieli O, Abramson A, Shacham R, et al. Endoscopic treatment of salivary gland injuries due to facial rejuvenation procedures. Laryngoscope 2008;118(5):763–7.

30. Nahlieli O, Baruchin AM. Sialoendoscopy: three years' experience as a diagnostic and treatment modality. J Oral Maxillofac Surg 1997;55(9):912–8.

31. Sionis S, Vedele A, Brennan PA, et al. Balloon catheter sialoplasty: a safety and feasibility pilot study. Br J Oral Maxillofac Surg 2013;51(3):228–30.

32. Ananthakrishnan N, Parkash S. Parotid fistulas: a review. Br J Surg 1982;69(11):641–3.

33. Motz KM, Kim YJ. Auriculotemporal syndrome (Frey syndrome). Otolaryngol Clin North Am 2016;49(2): 501–9.

34. Gomes-Ferreira PHS, de Carvalho Reis ENR, Faverani LP, et al. Frey syndrome after trauma: diagnosis and treatment. J Craniofac Surg 2017;28(2): 582–3.

35. Porcheri C, Mitsiadis TA. Physiology, pathology and regeneration of salivary glands. Cells 2019;8(9):976.

36. Yoshida S, Ohbo K, Takakura A, et al. Sgn1, a basic helix-loop-helix transcription factor delineates the salivary gland duct cell lineage in mice. Dev Biol 2001;240(2):517–30.

37. Bullard T, Koek L, Roztocil E, et al. Ascl3 expression marks a progenitor population of both acinar and ductal cells in mouse salivary glands. Dev Biol 2008;320(1):72–8.

Soft Tissue Trauma
Management of Lip Injury

Ashley Houle, DDS, MD[a,*], Michael R. Markiewicz, DDS, MD, MPH[b],
Nicholas Callahan, MPH, DMD, MD[a]

KEYWORDS

- Trauma • Lip injury • Lip laceration • Lip avulsion • Soft tissue injury • Management

KEY POINTS

- In-depth knowledge of lip anatomy will help a surgeon properly perform lip repair.
- Proper lip repair is key for the return of lip form and function.
- Correct alignment of the vermillion border is critical to an aesthetic repair.
- Local tissue arrangements are always preferred over distant donor sites for lip repair.

BACKGROUND: ANATOMY AND FUNCTION

The lips play a critical role in speech, nutritional intake, appearance, and sensation. Any injury and subsequent repair require consideration of these features and functions. The lips function as a muscular sphincter for the oral cavity, allowing for proper speech and swallowing without spillage of air or food from the oral cavity.[1,2]

The upper and lower lips are composed of several layers (from inside out) (**Fig. 1**)[3]:

- Mucosa
- Submucosa
- Muscle
- Subcutaneous fat
- Dermis
- Epidermis

The upper and lower lips receive vascular supply from branches of the facial artery, the superior and inferior labial arteries (**Fig. 2**A, B), respectively. Sensory information from the lips is carried by the infraorbital nerve and the inferior alveolar nerve (**Fig. 3**), which are branches of the trigeminal nerve. The facial nerve provides the motor innervation.[3,4]

Goals of management[4,5]

- Achieve 3-layered closure where indicated: mucosa, orbicularis oris, skin
- Restore the orbicularis oris sphincter
- Maintain the oral commissures when possible
- Maintain oral competence
- Maintain the size of the aperture (avoiding microstomia)
- Optimize esthetic outcome: continuity of the vermillion border, align vermillion border, the wet/dry line, and white roll, maintain appearance of philtral column and cupid's bow, symmetry, avoid distortion
- Minimize complications: infection, hematoma, scar formation, nerve injury

PATIENT EVALUATION OVERVIEW

A proper trauma workup must be performed to identify and manage any potentially life-threatening injuries in the primary survey. In the secondary survey, injury to the lips is addressed. A thorough history and physical examination should be performed to adequately assess the patient and avoid overlooking concurrent injuries. When indicated, appropriate imaging should be ordered and reviewed, particularly if there is concern of foreign body impaction in the soft tissues.[6] Pertinent components to the history and

[a] Department of Oral and Maxillofacial Surgery, University of Illinois at Chicago, 801 South Paulina, Room 110-DENT, Chicago, IL 60612, USA; [b] Department of Oral and Maxillofacial Surgery, University at Buffalo, 3425 Main Street, 112 Squire Hall, Buffalo, NY 14214, USA
* Corresponding author.
E-mail address: ahoule1@uic.edu

Oral Maxillofacial Surg Clin N Am 33 (2021) 351–357
https://doi.org/10.1016/j.coms.2021.04.003
1042-3699/21/© 2021 Elsevier Inc. All rights reserved.

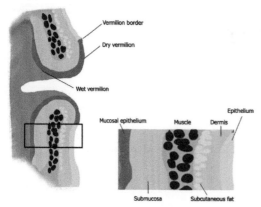

Fig. 1. Layers of the lip. Illustrations done by Dr Ashley Houle.

physical examination of the patient specific to addressing soft tissue trauma to the lips are listed in later discussion.[4,7,8]

- History
  - Mechanism
  - Associated symptoms
  - Age of wound
- Physical examination
  - Location
  - Extent of injury: depth, length, involvement of the vermillion border, layers involved (through-and-through laceration)
  - Condition of wound: gross contamination, foreign body impaction, such as an embedded tooth or fragment, devitalized tissue, hemostasis
  - Associated injuries (including underlying facial bone fractures)[9]

SURGICAL AND INTERVENTIONAL TREATMENT OPTIONS
Abrasion

An abrasion is a superficial wound typically caused by friction.[7] They tend to be quite painful, as terminal endings of nerve fibers are often involved. Minimal bleeding is encountered from superficial capillaries. When abrasions are superficial, there is typically minimal scarring. Thorough cleansing of the wound bed is indicated. If the abrasion is deep or foreign material and debris are noted, local anesthesia may be used for more aggressive scrubbing with a surgical brush and a petrolatum-based gel. It is imperative to remove all foreign debris at the time of initial injury before epidermal healing occurs. Aftercare includes the use of a topical antibiotic ointment with or without an overlying loose bandage. Petrolatum dressing changes may be used daily to cleanse the grossly contaminated wound. Abrasions to the mucosal lip often heal with no treatment. Chlorhexidine rinse may be given when gross contamination is present.

Puncture/Bite Wounds

Puncture and bite wounds often appear superficially small. However, care must be taken to appropriately cleanse and debride the area, as they can penetrate deeply. Deep penetration allows inoculation and embedding of bacteria, particularly with feline bite wounds. Closure is typically not indicated, as this can contribute to the development of infection. Bites from pit bulls are unique in that they tear tissue, causing avulsion and the need for additional reconstruction.

Contusion

Tissue disruption with subcutaneous or submucosal hemorrhage manifests as a contusion (bruise)[7] that typically does not involve a break in the surface tissues. The bleeding will tamponade when the hydrostatic pressure within the soft tissues equals the pressure within the blood vessels. Therefore, early intervention with ice and pressure dressing can aid in ceasing the bleed through vasoconstriction and pressure. Patients should be counseled regarding the ecchymosis expansion and progression of the contusion. Infection

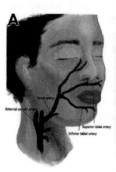
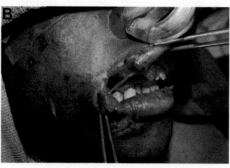

Fig. 2. (*A*) Vascular supply to the upper and lower lips. (*B*) Clinical image of intact labial artery after lip injury.

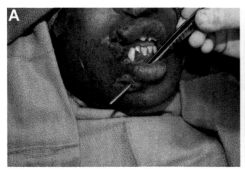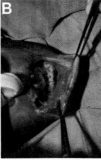

Fig. 3. (A) Through-and-through lip laceration with underlying mandible fracture. (B) Underlying mandibular fracture. The mental nerve can be visualized at the superior distal end of the mandibular hardware coursing to the laceration site.

is unlikely, and there is no indication for antibiotic therapy.

Laceration

Management of lip lacerations requires careful reapproximation of the involved layers so as to not compromise form and function.[4] Unlike surgical incisions, unfortunately one cannot control the design of a laceration. Understanding of the relaxed skin tension lines can help predict outcomes of closure (**Fig. 4**). Lacerations that cross perpendicular to the resting skin tension lines tend to widen and form a less esthetic scar. Therefore, it is crucial to provide good dermal support during closure, leaving no tension on the skin sutures. Most lacerations can be closed primarily, with the exception being in the setting of gross infection. In this situation, the wound may be packed with regular dressing changes and closed by delayed primary closure.

Before proceeding with the steps outlined in later discussion, it is important to achieve profound local anesthesia. Anesthetic blocks can be useful to avoid distortion of the area to be repaired.[10] Procedural sedation may be indicated in young or uncooperative children or complex lacerations requiring extensive revision and repair.

There are 4 major steps in the surgical management of a lip laceration. This approach applies to superficial lacerations, lacerations involving the vermilion border, and through-and-through lip lacerations (**Fig. 5**).[2,7]

- Cleansing/decontamination
  - Surgical soap and brush (petrolatum-based ointment to bring debris to superficial aspect of wound)
  - Saline to remove water-soluble material and flush out particulate matter
  - Pulse irrigation lavage has been shown to be superior to constant flow irrigation, but this can be difficult to perform in lip lacerations
  - Pressure irrigation with a 20-cc syringe and 18-gauge angiocath
- Debridement
  - Removal of contused and devitalized tissue, irregular pieces of tissue to enable linear closure, number 15 or 11 blade used to excise at right angles to skin and parallel to hair follicles
  - Hair at wound edges: clipped, not shaved

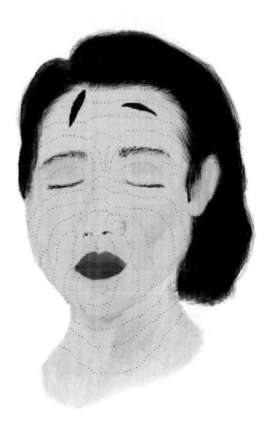

Fig. 4. Resting skin tension lines.

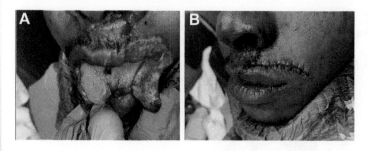

Fig. 5. (A) Incomplete avulsion of upper lip. (B) Closure of upper lip near avulsion.

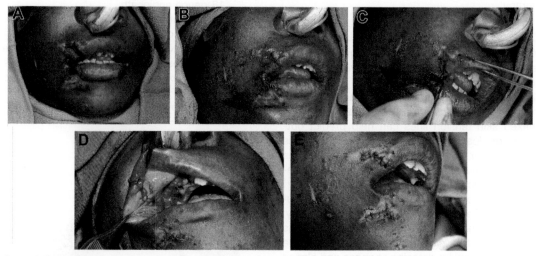

Fig. 6. (A) Complex lip laceration after motor vehicle accident. (B) Vermilion stitch. (C) Muscle layer closure. (D) Mucosal closure. (E) Final wound closure.

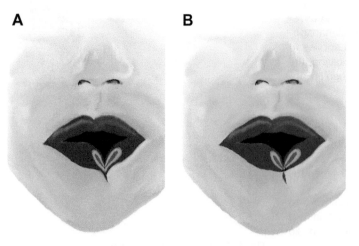

Fig. 7. Stay suture placed at vermillion border. (A) Lip laceration involving vermilion border. (B) First suture placed to reappoximate the vermilion border.

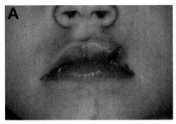
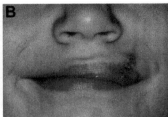

Fig. 8. (A) Laceration involving the vermilion border. (B) Primary repair with appropriate alignment of vermilion.

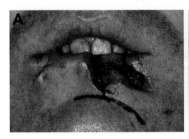
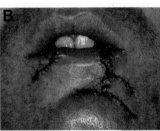

Fig. 9. (A) avulsion injury sustained by coyote bite with approximately one-third of lip defect. (B) Primary closure achieved with local advancement.

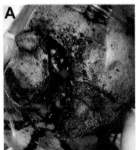
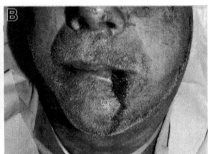

Fig. 10. (A) Extensive lip laceration on initial presentation; wound was temporized to allow for definite repair of facial fractures. (B) Approximately one-third of the lower lip was noted to be necrotic at time of facial bone repair.

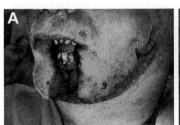
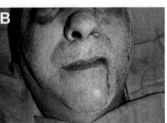

Fig. 11. (A) Wound after debridement of necrotic tissues. (B) Wound after primary closure of approximately one-third lip defect.

- Remove any obviously traumatized minor salivary glands
- Remove foreign material, can leave a traumatic tattoo, which is difficult to treat secondarily
- Hemostasis
  - Clamp and ligate large identifiable vessels with ligatures (or use monopolar or bipolar electrocautery)
  - Largest vessel encountered in lip laceration would be labial artery, approximately 1 mm in diameter, just under labial mucosa
- Closure
  - Location and depth impact manner in which wound is closed
  - Goal is to position all tissue layers properly with good muscle and dermal support
  - Any tension should be alleviated at the level of the reticular dermis

Small superficial lacerations involving only the wet vermilion or labial mucosa may not need to be closed. Larger lacerations, avulsed tissue or gaping wounds, or wounds with hemostasis issues can be closed with resorbable suture with buried knots (ie, 5-0 or 6-0 chromic gut suture).[4]

Superficial lacerations of the dry vermilion that do not involve the vermilion border are closed with resorbable suture in a simple interrupted fashion (5-0 or 6-0 chromic gut suture). If the vermillion border is involved, this is reapproximated first with a stay suture (6-0 nonabsorbable suture). The vermillion and oral mucosa should be closed with absorbable sutures, and skin should be closed with nonabsorbable sutures. If there is a concern regarding patient follow-up or for young children, fast-absorbing gut sutures may be substituted for nonabsorbable.[4]

Through-and-through lacerations require triple-layered closure. As with any laceration involving the vermillion border, this is reapproximated first with 6-0 Prolene or nylon. The laceration is then closed from the inside out.[2]

Recommendations

- Oral mucosa: resorbable suture such as chromic gut
- Orbicularis oris: interrupted resorbable sutures (braided or monofilament)
- Deep dermal sutures: interrupted resorbable sutures with buried knots
- Epidermis: 5-0 or 6-0 nylon or Prolene (monofilament) simple interrupted sutures
  - Needle should enter skin at a 90° angle and is approximately 2 mm away from the wound edge (atlas)

Sutures are to be removed within 4 to 6 days of placement. Adhesive strips may be placed at this time for external support (**Figs. 6–8**).

Avulsion

Avulsion injuries often result in portions of missing tissue.[4,7,8] Small defects may undergo direct repair, whereas intermediate defects may require recruitment of local flaps. Free tissue transfers may be indicated in the case of total or subtotal defects.

- Small defects: Direct repair
  - Upper lip defects up to one-fourth of lip
  - Lower lip defects up to one-third of lip
  - Goal of primary closure is to reestablish continuity of the orbicularis oris, allowing oral competence, maximum sensation preservation, continuity of the vermillion border, and adequate aperture size
  - See previous section on repair of lacerations for the proper management (**Figs. 9–12**)
- Intermediate defects: Local flaps
  - Abbe lip switch:
    - Often used to reconstruct defects due to avulsion injury or resection of pathologic condition.
    - Two-stage pedicled flap based on the labial artery
  - Estlander flap:
    - Triangular flap with lateral limb extending to the commissure
  - Bernard-Webster flap:
    - Advancement flap for lower lip reconstruction
  - Gillies fan flap:
    - Single-stage rotational advancement flap
    - Considered a modified or extended Estlander flap
  - Karapandzic flap:

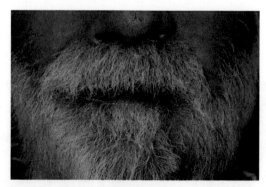

Fig. 12. Healing of lip wound at 2 months, showing good lip competence and esthetics.

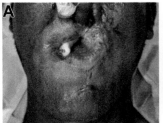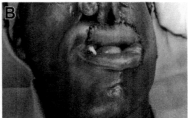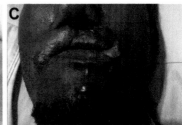

Fig. 13. (*A*) Patient with subtotal upper lip loss with loss of competency from a childhood injury. (*B*) Radial forearm used to rebuild the upper lip. (*C*) Patient at 6 months after repair, showing retention of upper lip competency.

- Axial musculo-mucocutaneous flap
- Partial thickness
- Total or subtotal defects: Free tissue (**Fig. 13**)

Aftercare and treatment adjuncts[11]

- Tetanus prophylaxis
- Antibiotics: systemic/topical
- Soft diet, avoid straws/spicy foods
- Remove sutures 4–6 days

SUMMARY

The lips play a critical role in speech, nutritional intake, appearance, and sensation. Any injury and subsequent repair require great consideration of these features and functions. This article reviews the common types of injury as well as management guidelines. Debridement and hemostasis are important before any formal repair, and this should be conducted with the patient's comfort considered, and whether intervention will require local versus general anesthesia. Goals of management include re-establishing form and function.

CLINICS CARE POINTS

- Achieve adequate local or general anesthesia before any debridement or repair but avoid distortion to the tissues.
- Align vermillion border first in lacerations involving this anatomic feature.
- Avoid tension superficially with a layered laceration closure.
- Understand relaxed skin tension lines.
- Avulsion injuries, depending on their extent, may require more advanced procedures for repair.

DISCLOSURE

The authors have nothing to disclose.

REFERENCES

1. Armstrong D. Lacerations of the mouth. Emerg Med Clin North America 2000;18(3):471–80.

2. Moskovitz JB, Sabatino F. Facial wound management. Emerg Med Clin North Am 2013;31(2):529–38.

3. Parlin LS. Repair of lip lacerations. Pediatr Rev 1997; 18(3):101–2.

4. Attia MW, Loiselle J. Management of soft-tissue injuries of the mouth. In: King C, Henretig FM, editors. Textbook of pediatric emergency procedures. 2nd edition. Philadelphia, PA: Lippincott, Williams & Wilkins; 2008. p. 680.

5. Nabili V, Knott PD. Advanced lip reconstruction: functional and aesthetic considerations. Facial Plast Surg 2008;24(1):092–104.

6. Lauritano D, Petruzzi M, Sacco G, et al. Dental fragment embedded in the lower lip after facial trauma: brief review literature and report of a case. Dental Res J 2012;9(2):237–41.

7. Ellis E III, Hupp JR, Tucker MR. Contemporary oral and maxillofacial surgery. St. Louis: Mosby-Year Book; 1993.

8. Kademani D, Tiwana P. Atlas of oral and maxillofacial surgery 2015. St Louis: Elsevier Health Sciences.

9. Antunes AA, Santos TS, Carvalho de Melo AU, et al. Tooth embedded in lower lip following dentoalveolar trauma: case report and literature review. Gen Dent 2012;60(6):544–7.

10. Moskovitz JB, Sabatino F. Regional nerve blocks of the face. Emerg Med Clin North Am 2013;31(2): 517–27.

11. Grunebaum LD, Smith JE, Hoosien GE. Lip and perioral trauma. Facial Plast Surg 2010;26(6): 433–44.

Fig. 13. (A) Patient with unfavorable upper lip loss of competency from a childhood injury. (B) Radial forearm used to rebuild the upper lip. (C) Patient at 6 months after repair, showing retention of upper lip competency.

- Axial muscle-mucocutaneous flap
- Radial forearm
- Local or distant islands: Free flaps (Fig. 13)

which are end treatment sub-entries:

- Healthy blood flaps
- Antibiotics systemic/topical
- Soft diet - avoid showy/spicy foods
- Remove sutures 4-5 days

SUMMARY

The lips play a crucial role in speech, nutritional intake, appearance, and sensation. Any injury (hard surface) that breaks great surfaces...

CLINICS CARE POINTS

- Address adequate level of general anesthesia before any management of repair that avoid distortion to the tissues.
- Approximate border first — landmarks involving this anatomic feature.
- Avoid trimming superficially with a layered laceration closure.
- Understand relaxed skin tension lines.
- Avulsion injuries, depending on their extent, may require more advanced procedures for repair.

REFERENCES

Updates in Management of Craniomaxillofacial Gunshot Wounds and Reconstruction of the Mandible

Baber Khatib, MD, DDS[a,b,c,*], Savannah Gelesko, MD, DDS[c],
Melissa Amundson, DDS[c,d], Allen Cheng, MD, DMD[c,d,e],
Ashish Patel, MD, DDS[c,d,f], Tuan Bui, MD, DDS[g], Eric J. Dierks, MD, DMD[c,d],
R. Bryan Bell, MD, DDS[c,d,f,h]

KEYWORDS

- Gunshot wounds • Mandible reconstruction • Facial trauma • Ballistic trauma
- Virtual surgical planning • Computer-aided surgery

KEY POINTS

- Mandibular injuries have been treated effectively for generations using closed reduction and open reduction with internal fixation.
- With advances in computer-aided surgery, complex and difficult surgeries are now possible with the precision and accuracy once achieved by only a select few seasoned surgeons.
- The increasing research and applications of custom hardware, patient-specific planning, and virtual surgery has led to, and will continue to lead to, improved patient function, improved esthetics, decreased operative times, decreased costs, and most importantly beneficial patient outcomes.

INTRODUCTION

Mandibular injuries have been treated effectively for generations using closed reduction and open reduction with internal fixation. Recently, there have been several notable advances in surgical management that have added substantially to a facial surgeon's ability to tackle simple as well as complex mandibular injuries more effectively.

Recent hardware advances in closed reduction include maxillomandibular fixation (MMF) screws in lieu of arch bars and hybrid systems that combine traditional arch bars with screw fixation. Open reduction and fixation has seen some very exciting applications of technology that include prebent and custom patient plates.

As a result of their complexity, treatment planning for facial ballistic injuries has seen an increase

This article originally appeared in November, 2017 issue of *Facial Plastic Surgery Clinics of North America* (Volume 25, Issue 4).
Disclosure statement: The authors have nothing to disclose.
[a] Advanced Craniomaxillofacial and Trauma Surgery/Head and Neck Oncologic and Microvascular Reconstructive Surgery, Department of Surgery, Legacy Emanuel Medical Center, 2801 N Gantentenbein Avenue, Portland, OR 97227, USA; [b] Providence Portland Hospital, 4805 NE Glisan Street, Portland, OR 97213, USA; [c] Head & Neck Surgical Associates, 1849 NW Kearney Street #302, Portland, OR 97209, USA; [d] Department of Surgery, Trauma Service, Legacy Emanuel Medical Center, 2801 N Gantentenbein Avenue, Portland, OR 97227, USA; [e] Head and Neck Cancer Program, Legacy Good Samaritan Medical Center, 1015 NW 22nd Avenue, Portland, OR 97210, USA; [f] Providence Oral, Head and Neck Cancer Program and Clinic, Providence Cancer Center, 4805 NE Glisan Street, Portland, OR 97213, USA; [g] Oral and Maxillofacial Pathology, Sanford Health, E - 1717 S University Drive Fargo, ND 58103, USA; [h] Robert W. Franz Cancer Research Center, Earle A. Chiles Research Institute at Providence Cancer Center, 4805 NE Glisan Street, Portland, OR 97213, USA
* Corresponding author. 1849 Northwest Kearney Street, #300, Portland, OR 97209.
E-mail address: baber.khatib@gmail.com

in the use of virtual surgery, patient-specific surgical guides, and intraoperative navigation and/or imaging to yield predictable and consistently repeatable results, once only achievable by seasoned surgeons.

The authors briefly review updates in management of mandibular trauma and reconstruction as they relate to MMF screws, custom hardware, virtual surgical planning (VSP), and protocols for use of computer-aided surgery and navigation when managing composite defects from gunshot injuries to the face.

Advances in Closed Reduction

MMF has a long history in the treatment of facial fractures dating back to 460 BC when Hippocrates used gold wire to fixate teeth for a mandible fracture.[1] Over the years there have been many modifications, including Barton bandage, suspension wires, Ivy loops, arch bars, MMF screws, and embrasure loops.[1–3] Erich arch bars (Karl Leibinger Co, Mulheim, Germany) continue to be the most commonly used technique. MMF screw fixation has the benefit of speedy application, decreased risk of puncture injury to the surgeon, less damage to the periodontium, and simple application and removal.[2,4–6] Their use is not without complications. The most commonly reported complications include screw loosening, iatrogenic damage to tooth roots, screw fracture, and ingestion.[7] A combination between MMF screws and arch bars known as *hybrid systems* are the newest advances to closed reduction. Commonly used systems include the SmartLock System Hybrid MMF (Stryker, Kalamazoo, MI), the MatrixWave (DePuy Synthes West Chester, PA), and the OmniMax MMF System (Zimmer Biomet, Jacksonville, FL). These systems are approved by the Food and Drug Administration for use in adults and children with fully erupted permanent dentition as a temporary means of fixation.[8–10] These systems allow expeditious placement associated with MMF screws while maintaining lugs at crown level, allowing traction vectors closer to the occlusal table. Potential complications are similar to those of MMF screws. Although the hybrid systems are much costlier than Erich arch bars, Kendrick and colleagues'[11] cost analysis of the Stryker SmartLock system versus traditional arch bars found no difference when accounting for operating room time, cost, and time saved.

Advances in Open Reduction

Virtual surgical planning/Stereolithography
Among the greatest technological advances in craniomaxillofacial (CMF) surgery is computer-aided CMF surgery. Bell[12] divides computer-aided CMF surgery into 3 main categories: (1) computer-aided presurgical planning, (2) intraoperative navigation, and (3) intraoperative computed tomography (CT)/MRI imaging. Computer-aided presurgical planning in mandibular trauma and reconstruction involves computer-aided design and computer-aided manufacturing (CAD/CAM) technology and VSP, which can then be applied to the fabrication of stereo-lithographic models and custom plates.[12–15]

Even in basic mandible fractures, intraoperative bending and contouring of reconstruction plates can be time consuming and inaccurate. Complex, multi-segment, and/or avulsed mandibular defects make this task much more difficult and potentially frustrating.

Although originally developed for industry, initial medical applications of CAD/CAM included neurosurgery and radiation therapy. CAD/CAM has since proven indispensable in the reconstruction of complex mandibular trauma and other CMF surgery.[16] CAD/CAM software enables the clinician to import 2-dimensional CT data in Digital Imaging and Communications in Medicine (DICOM) format to a computer workstation and to generate an accurate 3-dimensional (3D) representation of the skeletal and soft tissue anatomy. These digital models can be manipulated by virtual surgery allowing restoration of bony segments to their pretraumatic positions. Stereo-lithographic models of the virtually reduced mandible are then fabricated and can be used to manufacture custom cutting guides, plates, and splints.[12] These models have been reported to be accurate within 1 mm and have shown to decrease operative time and wound exposure time when used in the planning stage.[17,18]

Despite this degree of precision, there are a few areas where significant inaccuracies can be introduced. One critical area of inaccuracy is in the dental occlusion. CT scans, whether medical grade or cone beam, are unable to accurately capture occlusal anatomy. If accurate occlusal relationships are critical for surgical planning, then separate impressions must be taken from patients. These impressions can be done using traditional analog techniques with alginate/polyvinyl siloxane and stone or using newer digital impression techniques. Analog models are scanned into digital information. The dental and occlusal data can then be fused with the maxillofacial CT. Fusion can be done manually by a computer surgical planning engineer. However, if more precision is necessary, an occlusal fiduciary marker (a marker embedded in a bite registration or a bite registration mounted with a registration device) should be used when obtaining the maxillofacial CT and scanning the models. The fiduciary helps in accurately registering the models to the maxillofacial CT.

A second area of inaccuracy is in plate bending. The inherent rigidity of reconstruction plates makes them difficult to bend accurately, particularly when attempting to match the irregular contours of a mandible. Although smoothing osteoplasty can be performed on a model and subsequently transferred to patients, performing the same osteoplasty on patients potentially introduces another source of error. Repeated plate bending decreases fatigue resistance and increases the risk of plate fracture.[19,20] By combining the use of VSP, various CAD/CAM techniques, and novel surgical hardware manufacturing, it is now possible to implant custom plates that require little to no bending.

Custom plates

There are 3 main processes of manufacturing custom plates applicable to CMF surgery and mandible reconstruction: prebent plates, milled (subtractive manufacturing) plates, and additive layer manufacturing (ALM).

Prebent plates

In the infancy of stereo lithography (SLA), a well-documented technique involved printing a corrected stereo-lithographic model to which a reconstruction plate would be hand bent. Prebending decreases operative time and improves accuracy yet still introduces areas of fatigue more prone to failure with cyclic loading. Although the cause of plate fracture is multifactorial, limiting the number of bends to the plate should help maintain the original plate strength. The use of custom milled or printed plates substantially reduces the need for bending, often completely.

Subtractive and additive manufactured plates

The creation of milled plates is a subtractive technique that uses high-precision drills to cut a solid titanium/titanium alloy billet into the desired shape. Computer numerical control (CNC) machining dates back to the early 1940s when Parsons first created numerical control for the aerospace industry. CNC is the computer automation of machining tools, which eliminates the need for manual instrumentation. The 1940 CNC prototype engineered by Parsons at the Massachusetts Institute of Technology is the forebearer of this technology today.[21]

ALM, commonly known as 3D printing, is the newest technique used in plate fabrication. There are 2 main divisions within ALM: sintering and melting. Sintering involves heating metal powder to a temperature just before liquefaction, which allows cohesion to occur at the molecular level. This process allows control of porosity, which may later result in bone growth into the final structure. Melting involves the complete liquefaction of the metal within an accurately shaped container that results in a homogenous structure. These fabrication techniques are further divided into SLA, selective laser melting, selective laser sintering, and electron beam melting/direct metal printing. Current materials used in fracture and reconstruction plates include pure titanium and titanium, aluminum vanadium alloy (Ti6Al4V). Stainless steel 316L and cobalt chrome alloys have also been used in other applications.

Regardless of the additive method used, the basic steps are similar. A CT scan is taken after which the DICOM files are imported into a surgical planning software program. After the mandible is virtually reduced or reconstructed, the surgeon and the engineer collaborate, usually in the form of an online meeting, to design the plate. Once the final design is established, a software program slices the plate digitally into multiple horizontal layers. These data are then entered into a production machine that contains metal powder. A computer-guided laser runs over the powder and solidifies it layer by layer, from the bottom up. Any leftover powder can be reused, which is one major difference between ALM and milling. With milling, the shavings can be reused only after specialized processing, which is costly.

In both the subtractive and additive techniques, the plate is fully customizable and is designed over a digital workflow with an engineer and surgeon. Options for customization in both techniques include plate thickness, shape, screw hole position, number of screw holes, and varied thickness within the same reconstruction plate.

Navigation/intraoperative computed tomography

The digital workflow makes it possible to visualize the entire mandibular and facial skeleton, which is somewhat unrealistic. Unfortunately, these conditions do not translate directly to the operating room. Blood, edema, and avulsive soft and hard tissue defects can make it difficult to see appropriate landmarks for repair. A custom-fabricated plate that looks perfect during VSP can result in malocclusion, facial asymmetry, and poor bony adaptation if the implant does not seat in its exact planned position. The use of navigation systems has helped bridge the gap between virtual planning and reality.

As described by Bell,[12] navigation is analogous to global positioning systems (GPSs) in a car. The localizer represents a satellite in space; the instrument/probe represents track waves emitted by the GPS unit in the car; the preloaded CT scan represents the map.[12] Intraoperative navigation systems were initially developed for use in neurosurgery as a rigid system known as framed stereotaxy. Since its development, newer technology allows for navigation without rigid head frames, making the tool more accessible to other applications. Frameless stereotaxy is now used commonly in endoscopic surgery and in CMF surgery.[22–26] In CMF surgery, navigation is most commonly used in orbital reconstruction and has been reported to be accurate to within 1 to 2 mm.[27–29] By manipulating the surgical instrument affixed to a probe, one can precisely correlate a position on a computer surgically planned CT scan with patients in coronal, axial, and sagittal views. This ability allows for an intraoperative verification (evaluative phase) after the initial 3 phases of computer-aided CMF surgery have been completed (planning, modeling, surgery). The surgeon has the ability to adjust and verify in real time the positioning of bone and fixation, potentially avoiding an unnecessary return to the operating room if inconsistencies are seen on postoperative imaging.

Complex mandible reconstruction related to ballistic trauma

Gunshot wounds (GSWs) to the craniofacial region result in devastating functional disabilities and esthetic deformities, which are further magnified by the associated psychological trauma. Because most of these patients return to work, return to their preinjury lifestyle, and have a low rate of suicide recidivism, adequate reconstruction is essential to their comprehensive rehabilitation.[30,31]

Although most GSWs involve injuries to extremities, most self-inflicted GSWs are to the head and neck.[32] The infrequency of these injuries, combined with their enormous complexity, makes their reconstruction a daunting task. The complexity of these injuries prompted Rene Le Fort to exclude them in his classic article, reporting GSWs as "veritable explosions in the face" and "without surgical interest."[33] The reported mortality is 15%, with complications in those who survive as high as 30%.[34,35] Survivors have a long road to recovery that ideally involves a large multidisciplinary care team that includes surgeons, medicine, psychiatry, physical therapy, occupational therapy, speech/language pathology, case management, and social work.

In 2014, Shackford and colleagues[34] published an 11-year, 720-patient, multicenter retrospective review of GSW injuries to the face. Of the 720 patients, 20% died within 48 hours. Of those who survived the first 48 hours, 15% were ultimately discharged or transferred. The remaining 85% underwent surgical reconstruction. 41% of these injuries were the result of low-velocity handguns and 40% involved the mandible. Patients with mandibular trauma required an average of 1.7 operations. This finding was consistent with Taher's[36] review of 1135 facial gunshot injuries requiring an average of 1.5 operations.[34]

The tissue damage caused by high-velocity bullets (>1200 feet per second [fps], military/hunting weapons) results in tremendous soft and hard tissue defects both from immediate damage and progressive die-back phenomenon. Low-velocity bullets (<1200 fps) may not cause the same avulsive defects and rarely result in a significant die-back phenomenon but can result in comminution. Traditionally, external fixation was used in this setting to prevent further devascularization of bone secondary to periosteal stripping and to temporarily maintain large bony defects without soft tissue retraction until definitive repair. This procedure has been largely replaced with rigid internal fixation but is still a useful adjunct in the armamentarium for treatment of complex GSWs to the mandible. The significant defects caused by gunshot injuries to the mandible are not unlike those defects caused by ablative tumor surgery or necrotizing infection. Many of the techniques used in the reconstruction of ablative tumor defects can be applied to gunshot injuries to the mandible.

For those cases in which the soft tissue and hard tissue mandibular defects are amenable to primary repair, local flaps, and/or nonvascularized bone grafts, aided by VSP, can expedite the surgical process. In grossly comminuted fractures or continuity defects, the contralateral mandible can be mirrored to the injured side to approximate the mandible's pretraumatic form, which can then be used as described earlier to prebend plates or design custom plates.

The workflow starts with establishing stable reference points by placing patients in maxillomandibular fixation and taking a CT scan using the specific VSP protocol (typically 1-mm cuts) (www.medicalmodeling.com).[37] As mentioned earlier, stone models of the dentition can be sent to the surgical planning engineers and merged with the CT data for added accuracy. Next, a Web-based planning session is scheduled. The fractured and displaced bony segments are aligned virtually by an engineer guided by a surgeon. If any adjustments need to be made, they are done during the Web meeting. Once the virtual reduction has been completed and confirmed by the surgeon, the placement of the plate is virtually planned. If a custom plate is to be used, the surgeon can decide the shape of the plate, thickness (which can be varied across the length of the plate), and number of holes. Stereo-lithographic models are made to aid in reduction in the operating room. In some instances, positioning guides with predictive holes for the reconstruction plate can help with reduction. In segmental defects, cutting guides are made to precisely freshen the edges of the defects to allow for easy buttressing with reconstructed tissue (**Fig. 1**A–H).

For complex composite mandibular defects, microvascular reconstruction has become a mainstay. Ever since Hidalgo[38] reported the use of the fibula free flap for mandibular reconstruction, it has become the workhorse for such defects. Other flaps used in mandibular reconstruction include the deep circumflex iliac artery (DCIA) flap, scapula, and osteo-cutaneous radial forearm. For many reasons outside the scope of this article, the fibula flap is the most versatile and frequently used. The DCIA flap, scapula flap, and osteo-cutaneous radial forearm flaps have their specific indications but are used much less frequently in the authors' practice.[39]

There is some controversy over the method of fixation used for these reconstructions. Some investigators advocate fixation of the neo-mandible with mini-plates, whereas others prefer reconstruction plates.[38–41] Advocates of mini-plates argue that a stress-shielding phenomenon occurs with load-bearing reconstruction plates that impedes osseous healing. However, reconstruction plates have been shown to have less need for removal, lower infection rates, and greater ability to accurately shape the neo-mandible to mimic the native mandible.[41,42]

The mandible, when viewed from above, is shaped like an omega, with an irregular contour (**Fig. 2**). A common problem with adapting the fibula to the shape of the mandible is the discrepancy between the curved mandible and the straight fibula. Traditionally, multiple osteotomies were made to account for this discrepancy. However, recent cadaveric studies suggest that maintaining bone segments 2 cm or greater has a more reliable chance of containing a periosteal vessel then smaller segments (94% vs 65% in 1.0 cm).[43] One method to address the discrepancy, while also limiting the number of fibula osteotomies required, is to take a subunit approach to mandibular reconstruction. The mandibular defect is divided into subunits (body, symphysis, condyle, and ramus). Fibula osteotomies are performed allowing for a straight segment to replace each of these subunits, as necessary. Therefore, a hemi-mandibular defect would only require 2

closing osteotomies and 3 segments, each with sufficient length to maintain vascularity. In addition, this simplifies adaptation of the reconstructive plate to the neo-mandible.

Early on, a stereo-lithographic model could be made by mirroring the contralateral mandible and ground to a flat surface, simulating the fibula. Now, data from stock fibulas can be loaded into the surgical planning software, which can then be printed directly into the stereo-lithographic model for prebending. Alternatively, patient-specific fibula data taken from CT angiograms of the extremities can be loaded into the surgical planning software, for greater accuracy.

In addition, computer-aided surgical planning allows accurate reconstruction in 3 dimensions.[15] Establishing the correct transverse, anterior-posterior, and vertical dimension of the lower face, while simultaneously positioning the neo-mandible to the opposing dental arch at the correct vertical dimension of occlusion, used to be incredibly difficult with the limitations of our surgical approaches to the facial skeleton. Now, this accurate positioning in 3 dimensions is easily verified using virtual models and replicated intraoperatively using guides, navigation, and/or intraoperative CT. These techniques have proven to be accurate, cost saving, and efficient.[44–46] Furthermore, these techniques allow for more predictable implant supported prosthetic rehabilitation while preventing overprojection of the mandible.[12]

Much of the bench work has been moved to the virtual realm with advances in CAD/CAM software and additive manufacturing of surgical guides and custom plates. In 2009, Hirsch and colleagues[47] described the use of Surgi Case CMF software (Materialise, Leuven, Belgium) to virtually plan a mandibular resection and reconstruction with a free fibula flap. The virtually planned osteotomies were incorporated into a surgical guide designed using planning software, then manufactured using a 3D printer, thereby transferring the virtual plan into an intraoperative tool. These surgical guides were then used to create the virtually planned osteotomies in vivo (Medical Modeling, Inc, Golden, CO). This practice allowed the vascularized composite tissue to reconstruct the mandible with ideal anterior/posterior, vertical, and transverse positioning. Levine and colleagues[48] and Hirsch and colleagues[47] have taken this a step further, developing a protocol for Jaw in a Day. In this protocol, they are able to virtually plan a mandibular segmental resection, reconstruction with a fibula free flap, guided placement of dental implants into the fibula, and a fixed provisional hybrid prosthesis that is immediately placed and

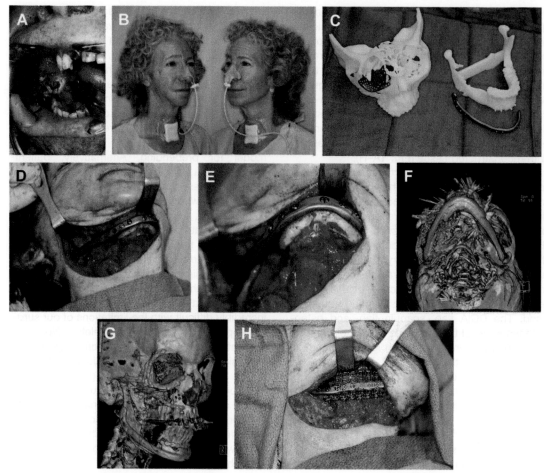

Fig. 1. (A–G): A 54-year-old woman with self-inflicted GSW to the face resulting in a segmental defect of the right mandibular body and orbital floor fracture reconstructed with custom orbital floor plate and mandibular reconstruction plate. Segmental defect grafted with autogenous iliac crest, platelet rich plasma (PRP), and bone morphogenetic protein (BMP). (A) Intraoral photograph showing comminution of right mandible. (B) One month after MMF, tracheostomy, debridement, wound closure, and feeding tube placement. (C) Custom printed mandibular reconstruction plate and orbital floor plate on stereo-lithographic models. (D) Custom mandibular reconstruction plate in situ. (E) Intimate adaptation of custom mandibular reconstruction plate. (F) Axial view of facial CT with plate in place. (G) The 3D reconstruction of CT with custom hardware in place. (H) Autogenous iliac bone graft/PRP/BMP in titanium mesh 3 months after initial injury.

loaded, all in one surgery.[48] This procedure has been successfully replicated at several institutions, including the authors' own. It has allowed surgeons to take patients to premorbid form and function in 1 day, an end point that previously would require 1 or more years.[49,50] This concept could be applied to mandibular traumatic defects.

Composite mandibular defects can also be managed with the use of distraction osteogenesis (DO). The technique was first described for mandibular reconstruction in 1920 by Rosenthal but did not become popularized until the Ilizarov protocols on limb DO in 1951.[51] It proved advantageous for reconstruction of the facial skeleton in its ability to address both hard and soft tissue

deficiencies. A common difficulty associated with this technique is the unpredictable control of the regenerative chamber vector. With stock distraction prostheses, a set linear trajectory is built into the prosthesis dictated by the screw. Bidirectional screws, endless screws, and multi-planar 3D distraction have been described; however, their application to GSW injuries is limited by the inability to locate precise anatomic landmarks.[52,53]

With the advent of computer surgical planning, DO is once again a useful tool in the reconstructive armamentarium. Benateau and colleagues[54] described the use of computer-assisted custom distraction devices and cutting guides for reconstruction of the lower face after gunshot injury.[54]

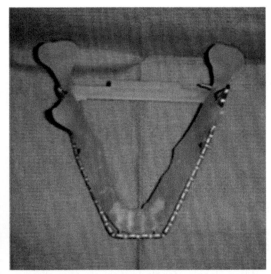

Fig. 2. Omega shape of mandible versus straight fibula.

Similar to computer surgical planning discussed earlier, planning for DO facilitates management of the spatial position of the neo-mandible in reference to the dentition and occlusal plane of the maxilla. Akin to the authors' experience with self-inflicted mandible GSW injures, Benateau and colleagues[54] found the ramus/condyle unit tends to be spared. The segments were repositioned virtually; osteotomy lines were planned; and predictive markers were used on the cutting guides for placement of the distraction device. The 2 cases reported showed excellent symmetry and reconstruction of an 8.5-cm and 10.0-cm defect.

In comparison with fibula free flaps, Wojcik and colleagues[55] showed that there was less cost associated with standard DO because of the shorter hospitalization these procedures required. Even though the overall duration of treatment was longer, the duration of hospitalization was shorter on average by 10 days.[55] Another point to consider is the impact of failed therapy. The morbidity associated with failed distraction is significantly less than that of a failed fibula, with the added drawback of donor site morbidity. Nonetheless, case selection is important and the fibula free flap remains the workhorse for reconstruction of composite mandibular defects.

Protocol for Computer-Aided Surgical Reconstruction of Massive Craniomaxillofacial Gunshot Wounds: Focus on Composite Mandibular Defects

At the authors' institution, patients are initially evaluated and managed in accordance to the advance trauma life support system (**Fig. 3**). Particular importance is placed on the airway, as bleeding into the tight compartmentalized spaces of the neck, avulsion of the tongue's attachments, tongue edema, blood, bone, debris, and foreign objects can result in rapidly progressive airway compromise. Oral intubation is often successful with few patients requiring emergent cricothyrotomy or tracheostomy. This finding is consistent with Shackford and colleagues'[34] and Demetriades and colleagues'[35] studies, which reported 83% of patients with facial GSWs were successfully orally intubated and only 5% required a surgical airway.[34,35] Once patients are stabilized, an elective tracheostomy is performed for definitive airway management for the reconstruction phase. A thorough head and neck examination is performed in conjunction with the primary and secondary survey. In patients with penetrating neck injury, the authors follow a selective neck exploration protocol.[56] Those with hard signs of vascular injury, including expanding hematoma, massive subcutaneous emphysema, exsanguinating hemorrhage, shock, or airway compromise, and those with respiratory and hemodynamic stability with violation of the platysma and positive computer angiography tomography (CTA) findings warrant surgical exploration (**Fig. 5**A).

After patients are stabilized, they are taken for debridement, damage control surgery, elective tracheostomy, and feeding tube placement often the same day as arrival. This practice involves washout of the wound, examination under anesthesia (direct laryngoscopy, rigid esophagoscopy and/or esophagogastroduodenoscopy) surgical hemostasis, conservative debridement of frankly necrotic tissues, and wound closure and/or packing. Occasionally, some bony fixation may be applied, if it can be done easily and quickly. The primary objective is to achieve control of the wound and perform an initial assessment. During the time immediately after injury, while patients are marginally stable and in a profound inflammatory state, extended and lengthy procedures should be avoided. Damage control surgeries may require daily short trips to the operating room, particularly with evolving injuries, as is seen in ballistics or burn injuries (see **Fig. 5**B–D).

At this point, a maxillofacial CT scan with 1-mm fine cuts is taken. If a fibula flap is required, a CT angiogram of the lower extremities is also taken. The data are uploaded to the surgical planning software. The maxillofacial surgery team then schedules a Web meeting with an engineer to virtually plan the reconstructions.

The authors' goal is to complete as much of the skeletal and soft tissue reconstruction as possible

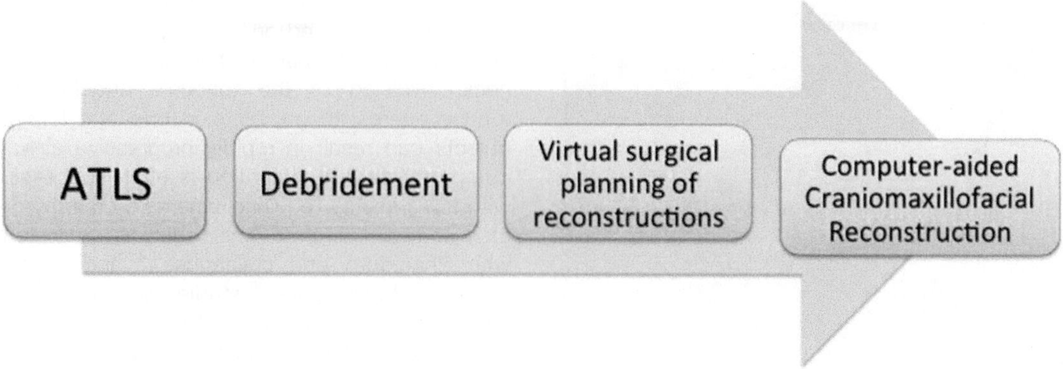

ATLS → Debridement → Virtual surgical planning of reconstructions → Computer-aided Craniomaxillofacial Reconstruction

Fig. 3. CMF GSW protocol. ATLS, advanced trauma life support.

during the initial hospitalization, with the understanding that revisions will certainly occur later. The authors prefer to stage the computer-aided CMF reconstruction in the following sequence (**Fig. 4**).

The authors begin with the midfacial and orbital reconstruction because of their importance in establishing proper facial width. A reciprocal relationship exists between anterior-posterior projection of the zygoma and facial width. By straightening the zygomatic arch, zygoma projection increases with a resultant decrease in facial width.[57] Stereo-lithographic models are created after virtually reducing midfacial fractures and plates are contoured to them intraoperatively. Intraoperative navigation facilitates accurate reduction and fixation (**Fig. 5E–H**).

Once the bizygomatic width is established, the authors focus on oromandibular reconstruction. The authors find that in self-inflicted GSWs, the condyle ramus unit tends to be spared. This preservation facilitates establishing the vertical dimension of the lower face against the already established transverse width by virtually seating the condyles in the fossa. Composite defects are then reconstructed with a fibula and custom

reconstruction plate or custom plate alone in the case of adequate soft tissue and bone for a non-vascularized bone grafts (see **Fig. 1D**).

When planning for fibula reconstruction, the authors prefer butt joints between native mandible and reconstruction to facilitate flap inset. These butt joints are virtually created at the junction of reconstructive subunits (see **Fig. 5I**). Attention is then drawn to the 3D virtual fibula created from preloaded CTA data of the lower extremity.

Depending on the location of recipient vessels in the neck, location of the soft tissue defect and the need for anterior versus posterior positioning of the pedicle the ipsilateral or contralateral fibula is used. For body defects, body and symphysis defects, or angle to angle defects with ipsilateral recipient vessels available, the authors typically have the vessels run posterior. When the condylar ramus subunit needs to be reconstructed, the authors prefer vessels run anteriorly as this mitigates the need for hairpins in the vessels around the skull base. The engineer then virtually performs a distal osteotomy 6 to 7 cm from the malleolus and closing osteotomies to allow the defect to be filled from posterior to anterior restoring each missing subunit (see **Fig. 5J**). The remaining bone on the

Fig. 4. CMF GSW reconstruction protocol.

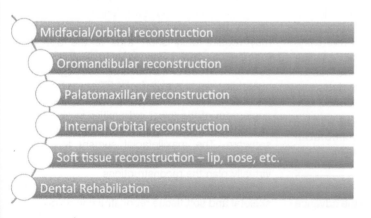

Midfacial/orbital reconstruction

Oromandibular reconstruction

Palatomaxillary reconstruction

Internal Orbital reconstruction

Soft tissue reconstruction – lip, nose, etc.

Dental Rehabiliation

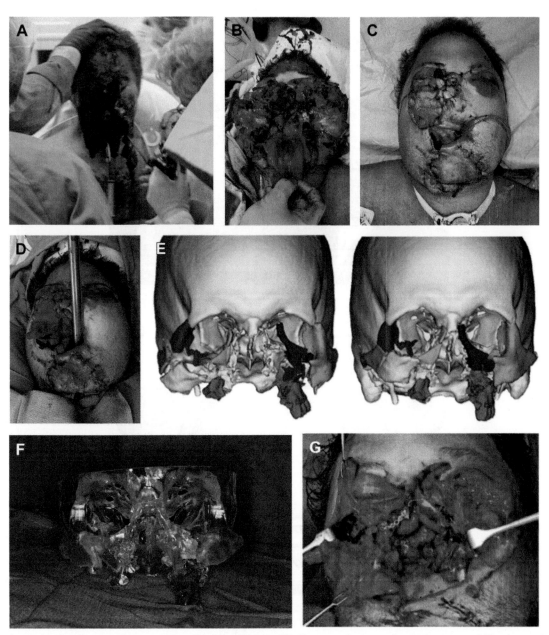

Fig. 5. (*A–P*) A 30-year-old man with self-inflicted GSW with 12-gauge shotgun who underwent stabilization and staged reconstruction following the authors' protocol. (*A*) Patient orally intubated and being stabilized by advanced trauma life support protocol. (*B*) Wound exploration, washout, conservative debridement, tracheostomy. (*C*) Wound closure, damage control. (*D*) Rigid esophagoscopy, direct laryngoscopy. (*E*) Virtual reduction of nasoorbitalethmoidal (NOE) and Le Fort III fractures. (*F*) Stereo-lithographic model with reduced NOE/Le Fort III fractures. (*G*) Open feeding gastrostomy tube placement, open reduction internal fixation Le Fort III fractures, NOE fractures, medial canthopexy. (*H*) Intraoperative navigation facilitates transfer of virtual plan to operating room. (*I*) Virtual surgical cutting guides to create butt joints at native mandible fibula junction. (*J*) Virtual planning of fibula osteotomies. (*K*) Fibula is placed intermediately between alveolus and inferior border at body region. (*L*) Left to right: mandible cutting guide, stereo-lithographic native mandible/maxilla (*pink*), neomandible model (*white*) with custom reconstruction plate. (*M*) Cutting guides on fibula (*top*) mandible (*bottom*). (*N*) Fibula inset with perfect adaptation of custom reconstruction plate. (*O*) Virtual planning for maxilla reconstruction with a fibula. (*P*) Use of intraoperative navigation during maxillary reconstruction.

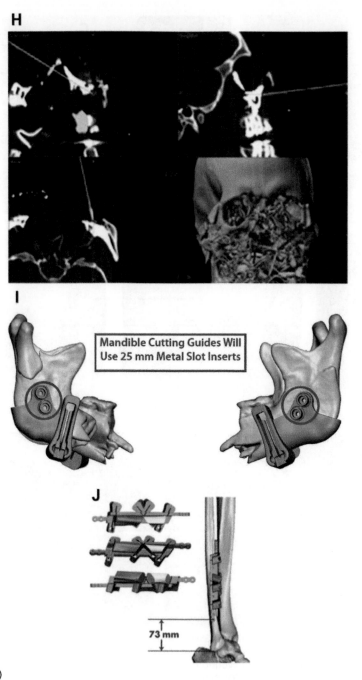

Fig. 5. (*continued*)

proximal fibula is removed and represents pedicle length. The authors choose to place the fibula at an intermediate point between the alveolus and inferior border of the mandible when reconstructing the body and at the inferior border and slightly lateral for reconstruction of the angle. This location allows for ideal placement of dental implants under the maxillary alveolus, providing adequate soft

tissue for closure while still maintaining facial symmetry and facial contour (see **Fig. 5**K).

After this reconstructive planning phase, the engineer-surgeon team designs cutting guides and 3D prints them for use intraoperatively. The mandibular cutting guides are fixated on the lateral native mandible with mono-cortical screws and include a removable metal insert allowing for saw

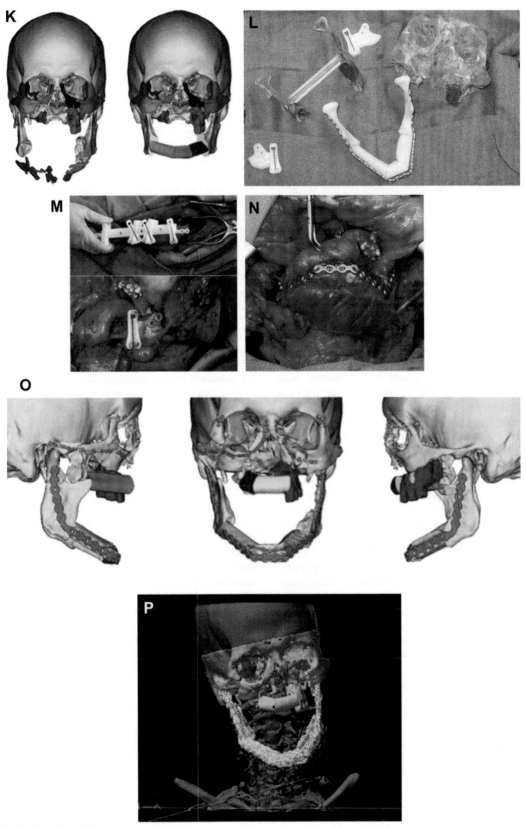

Fig. 5. (*continued*)

placement at the osteotomy site. Predictive holes are made that facilitate placement of the custom reconstruction plate. The fibula cutting guide is preferentially designed to rest on the lateral side of the fibula, which aids in protection of the pedicle during osteotomies and with a 0.5-mm relief to account for soft tissue. A mark is placed on the cutting guide to designate an arbitrarily selected distance from the lateral malleolus, to aid in fitting the fibula guide at the appropriate position along the proximal-distal axis. Finally, a custom 3D-printed reconstruction plate is engineered that matches predictive holes placed on the surgical guides. Templates are also fabricated of the bone graft and plate to assure the actual osteotomies match the computer-simulated plan. Lastly, the VSP data are merged with the original CT scan and overlaid for use with intraoperative navigation (see **Fig. 5**I, L).

Intraoperatively, a 2-team approach is used: one to perform the mandibular osteotomies, place the custom reconstruction plate, and locate recipient vessels while the second team harvests the fibula and shapes it to the computer-aided surgical plan (see **Fig. 5**M). The fibula is then inset, and the microvascular anastomosis is completed (see **Fig. 5**N). If the lip is being reconstructed with the soft tissue pedicle, a tensor fascia lata sling is suspended from the maxilla with Mitek mini anchors (Mitek Products Inc, Westwood, MA). The reconstruction is compared with planned reconstruction with bone graft templates and intraoperative navigation. At the completion of this phase, a postoperative CT scan is taken for the next phase of VSP.

Palatomaxillary reconstruction follows a subunit protocol similar to Brown and colleagues'[58] classification and Bell's[12] VSP approach. If composite reconstruction is planned, the digital workflow is similar to fibula reconstruction of the mandible. Reconstruction of maxilla in the correct 3D orientation is limited by accessibility and visibility in a confined space. An area of particular difficulty is abutting the fibula to the pterygoid plates, which can result in widening and a cant of the maxilla. Intraoperative navigation is an indispensable tool in this aspect. Other reconstructive options include the scapula tip or anterior lateral thigh/radial forearm for soft tissue only (see **Fig. 5**O, P).

Internal orbital reconstruction begins by comparing the internal orbital volume measured by the computer planning engineer. Virtual correction is then made using the uninjured or anatomically correct side by creating a mirror image that superimposes the traumatized side. In bilateral fractures, the least comminuted orbit is virtually corrected and then mirror imaged to the contralateral side. Custom orbital plates and/or stereo-lithographic models are then fabricated using the virtually corrected orbits. With stereo-lithographic models, a mesh plate is contoured preoperatively. Intraoperatively, the plates are positioned with the aid of navigation to locate the posterior orbital ledge. Navigation is then used to confirm its position in relation to the computer-simulated plan in the following sequential systematic protocol: malar eminence, infraorbital rim, lateral orbital rim, orbital floor, medial internal orbit/posteromedial orbital bulge, lateral internal orbit, posterior orbit/orbital apex, and finally globe projection. The authors find this technique reliably establishes orbital contour, volume, anterior bulge, and posterior medial bulge.[12,59–62]

Following a period of healing and establishment of a bony foundations, patients then undergo soft tissue reconstruction. Soft tissue procedures include rotational flaps, fat grafts, injectable fillers, and magnetic implant–supported prosthesis and are beyond the scope of this article.

Lastly, dental rehabilitation and reconstruction of a functional occlusion are performed. This process involves dental implants, hybrid prosthesis fabrication, and communication between the facial surgeon and the prosthodontist.

With this protocol, the authors find they get the best chance of establishing proper facial width, projection, and contour to produce a functional and reasonably esthetic facial reconstruction.

SUMMARY

With advances in computer-aided surgery, complex and difficult surgeries are now possible with the precision and accuracy once achieved by only a select few seasoned surgeons. The increasing research and applications of custom hardware, patient-specific planning, and virtual surgery has led to, and will continue to lead to, improved patient function, improved esthetics, decreased operative times, decreased costs, and most importantly beneficial patient outcomes.

REFERENCES

1. Mukerji R, Mukerji G, McGurk M. Mandibular fractures: historical perspective. Br J Oral Maxillofac Surg 2006;44(3):222–8.

2. Hollows P, Brennan J. Temporary intermaxillary fixation: a quick reliable method. Br J Oral Maxillofac Surg 1999;37(5):422–3.

3. Karlis V, Glickman R. An alternative to arch-bar maxillomandibular fixation. Plast Reconstr Surg 1997; 99(6):1758–9.

4. Arthur G, Berardo N. A simplified technique of maxillomandibular fixation. J Oral Maxillofac Surg 1989; 47(11):1234.

5. Onishi K, Maruyama Y. Simple intermaxillary fixation for maxillomandibular osteosynthesis. J Craniofac Surg 1996;7(2):170–2.

6. Schneider AM, David LR, DeFranzo AJ, et al. Use of specialized bone screws for intermaxillary fixation. Ann Plast Surg 2000;44(2):154–7.

7. Hashemi HM, Parhiz A. Complications using intermaxillary fixation screws. J Oral Maxillofac Surg 2011;69(5):1411–4.

8. DePuy synthes FDA approval. Available at: https://www.accessdata.fda.gov/cdrh_docs/pdf14/K141165.pdf. Accessed January 11, 2016.

9. Stryker Corp. Stryker craniomaxillofacial. Available at: http://www.accessdata.fda.gov/cdrh_docs/pdf12/K122313.pdf. Accessed January 11, 2016.

10. 510K Summary_Revised_12-10-2015-FDA. Available at: https://www.accessdata.fda.gov/cdrh_docs/pdf15/K152326.pdf. Accessed January 11, 2016.

11. Kendrick DE, Park CM, Fa JM, et al. Stryker SMART-Lock hybrid maxillomandibular fixation system: clinical application, complications, and radiographic findings. Plast Reconstr Surg 2016;137(1):142e–50e.

12. Bell RB. Computer planning and intraoperative navigation in cranio-maxillofacial surgery. Oral Maxillofac Surg Clin North Am 2010;22(1):135–56.

13. Bell RB, Weimer KA, Dierks EJ, et al. Computer planning and intraoperative navigation for palatomaxillary and mandibular reconstruction with fibular free flaps. J Oral Maxillofac Surg 2011;69(3):724–32.

14. Bui TG, Bell RB, Dierks EJ. Technological advances in the treatment of facial trauma. Atlas Oral Maxillofac Surg Clin North Am 2012;20(1):81–94.

15. Markiewicz MR, Bell RB. The use of 3D imaging tools in facial plastic surgery. Facial Plast Surg Clin North Am 2011;19(4):655–82, ix.

16. Schramm A, Wilde F. Computer-assisted reconstruction of the facial skeleton. HNO 2011;59(8):800–6 [in German].

17. Barker TM, Earwaker WJ, Lisle DA. Accuracy of stereolithographic models of human anatomy. Australas Radiol 1994;38(2):106–11.

18. Mehra P, Miner J, D'Innocenzo R, et al. Use of 3-d stereolithographic models in oral and maxillofacial surgery. J Maxillofac Oral Surg 2011;10(1):6–13.

19. Martola M, Lindqvist C, Hänninen H, et al. Fracture of titanium plates used for mandibular reconstruction following ablative tumor surgery. J Biomed Mater Res B Appl Biomater 2007;80(2):345–52.

20. Alberts LR, Phillips KO, Tu HK, et al. A biologic model for assessment of osseous strain patterns and plating systems in the human maxilla. J Oral Maxillofac Surg 2003;61(1):79–88.

21. History of CNC milling and turning machines. Available at: http://www.cam-machine.com/history-of-cnc-milling-and-turning-machines/. Accessed June 11, 2016.

22. Hassfeld S, Muhling J. Computer assisted oral and maxillofacial surgery–a review and an assessment of technology. Int J Oral Maxillofac Surg 2001; 30(1):2–13.

23. Drake JM, Joy M, Goldenberg A, et al. Computer- and robot-assisted resection of thalamic astrocytomas in children. Neurosurgery 1991;29(1):27–33.

24. Mosges R, Klimek L. Computer-assisted surgery of the paranasal sinuses. J Otolaryngol 1993;22(2): 69–71.

25. Ossoff RH, Reinisch L. Computer-assisted surgical techniques: a vision for the future of otolaryngology-head and neck surgery. J Otolaryngol 1994;23(5):354–9.

26. Barnett GH. Surgical management of convexity and falcine meningiomas using interactive image-guided surgery systems. Neurosurg Clin N Am 1996;7(2): 279–84.

27. Metzger MC, Rafii A, Holhweg-Majert B, et al. Comparison of 4 registration strategies for computer-aided maxillofacial surgery. Otolaryngol Head Neck Surg 2007;137(1):93–9.

28. Luebbers HT, Messmer P, Obwegeser JA, et al. Comparison of different registration methods for surgical navigation in cranio-maxillofacial surgery. J Craniomaxillofac Surg 2008;36(2):109–16.

29. Austin RE, Antonyshyn OM. Current applications of 3-d intraoperative navigation in craniomaxillofacial surgery: a retrospective clinical review. Ann Plast Surg 2012;69(3):271–8.

30. Ozturk S, Bozkurt A, Durmus M, et al. Psychiatric analysis of suicide attempt subjects due to maxillofacial gunshot. J Craniofac Surg 2006;17(6):1072–5.

31. Shuck LW, Orgel MG, Vogel AV. Self-inflicted gunshot wounds to the face: a review of 18 cases. J Trauma 1980;20(5):370–7.

32. Cunningham LL, Haug RH, Ford J. Firearm injuries to the maxillofacial region: an overview of current thoughts regarding demographics, pathophysiology, and management. J Oral Maxillofac Surg 2003;61(8):932–42.

33. Tessier P. The classic reprint. Experimental study of fractures of the upper jaw. I and II. Rene Le Fort, M.D. Plast Reconstr Surg 1972;50(5):497–506 contd.

34. Shackford SR, Kahl JE, Calvo RY, et al. Gunshot wounds and blast injuries to the face are associated with significant morbidity and mortality: results of an 11-year multi-institutional study of 720 patients. J Trauma Acute Care Surg 2014;76(2):347–52.

35. Demetriades D, Chahwan S, Gomez H, et al. Initial evaluation and management of gunshot wounds to the face. J Trauma 1998;45(1):39–41.

36. Taher AA. Management of weapon injuries to the craniofacial skeleton. J Craniofac Surg 1998;9(4): 371–82.

37. 3D systems cranio-maxillofacial CT scanning protocol. Available at: http://www.medicalmodeling.com/downloads. Accessed November 6, 2016.

38. Hidalgo DA. Fibula free flap: a new method of mandible reconstruction. Plast Reconstr Surg 1989;84(1):71–9.

39. Disa JJ, Cordeiro PG. Mandible reconstruction with microvascular surgery. Semin Surg Oncol 2000; 19(3):226–34.

40. Hidalgo DA, Pusic AL. Free-flap mandibular reconstruction: a 10-year follow-up study. Plast Reconstr Surg 2002;110(2):438–49 [discussion: 450–1].

41. Bell RB, Dierks EJ, Potter JK, et al. A comparison of fixation techniques in oro-mandibular reconstruction utilizing fibular free flaps. J Oral Maxillofac Surg 2007;65(9):39.

42. Al-Bustani S, Austin GK, Ambrose EC, et al. Miniplates versus reconstruction bars for oncologic free fibula flap mandible reconstruction. Ann Plast Surg 2016;77(3):314–7.

43. Fry AM, Laugharne D, Jones K. Osteotomising the fibular free flap: an anatomical perspective. Br J Oral Maxillofac Surg 2016;54(6):692–3.

44. Toto JM, Chang EI, Agag R, et al. Improved operative efficiency of free fibula flap mandible reconstruction with patient-specific, computer-guided preoperative planning. Head Neck 2015;37(11): 1660–4.

45. Metzler P, Geiger EJ, Alcon A, et al. Three-dimensional virtual surgery accuracy for free fibula mandibular reconstruction: planned versus actual results. J Oral Maxillofac Surg 2014;72(12):2601–12.

46. Weijs WL, Coppen C, Schreurs R, et al. Accuracy of virtually 3D planned resection templates in mandibular reconstruction. J Craniomaxillofac Surg 2016; 44(11):1828–32.

47. Hirsch DL, Garfein ES, Christensen AM, et al. Use of computer-aided design and computer-aided manufacturing to produce orthognathically ideal surgical outcomes: a paradigm shift in head and neck reconstruction. J Oral Maxillofac Surg 2009;67(10): 2115–22.

48. Levine JP, Bae JS, Soares M, et al. Jaw in a day: total maxillofacial reconstruction using digital technology. Plast Reconstr Surg 2013;131(6):1386–91.

49. Qaisi M, Kolodney H, Swedenburg G, et al. Fibula jaw in a day: state of the art in maxillofacial reconstruction. J Oral Maxillofac Surg 2016;74(6):1284. e1–15.

50. Monaco C, Stranix JT, Avraham T, et al. Evolution of surgical techniques for mandibular reconstruction using free fibula flaps: the next generation. Head Neck 2016;38(Suppl 1):E2066–73.

51. Cope JB, Samchukov ML, Cherkashin AM. Mandibular distraction osteogenesis: a historic perspective and future directions. Am J Orthod Dentofacial Orthop 1999;115(4):448–60.

52. Labbe D, Nicolas J, Kaluzinski E, et al. Gunshot wounds: two cases of midface reconstruction by osteogenic distraction. J Plast Reconstr Aesthet Surg 2009;62(9):1174–80.

53. Gateno J, Teichgraeber JF, Aguilar E. Distraction osteogenesis: a new surgical technique for use with the multiplanar mandibular distractor. Plast Reconstr Surg 2000;105(3):883–8.

54. Benateau H, Chatellier A, Caillot A, et al. Computer-assisted planning of distraction osteogenesis for lower face reconstruction in gunshot traumas. J Craniomaxillofac Surg 2016;44(10):1583–91.

55. Wojcik T, Ferri J, Touzet S, et al. Distraction osteogenesis versus fibula free flap for mandibular reconstruction after gunshot injury: socioeconomic and technical comparisons. J Craniofac Surg 2011; 22(3):876–82.

56. Bell RB, Osborn T, Dierks EJ, et al. Management of penetrating neck injuries: a new paradigm for civilian trauma. J Oral Maxillofac Surg 2007;65(4): 691–705.

57. Gruss JS, Van Wyck L, Phillips JH, et al. The importance of the zygomatic arch in complex midfacial fracture repair and correction of posttraumatic orbitozygomatic deformities. Plast Reconstr Surg 1990; 85(6):878–90.

58. Brown JS, Shaw RJ. Reconstruction of the maxilla and midface: introducing a new classification. Lancet Oncol 2010;11(10):1001–8.

59. Bell RB, Markiewicz MR. Computer-assisted planning, stereolithographic modeling, and intraoperative navigation for complex orbital reconstruction: a descriptive study in a preliminary cohort. J Oral Maxillofac Surg 2009;67(12):2559–70.

60. Markiewicz MR, Dierks EJ, Bell RB. Does intraoperative navigation restore orbital dimensions in traumatic and post-ablative defects? J Craniomaxillofac Surg 2012;40(2):142–8.

61. Markiewicz MR, Dierks EJ, Potter BE, et al. Reliability of intraoperative navigation in restoring normal orbital dimensions. J Oral Maxillofac Surg 2011; 69(11):2833–40.

62. Markiewicz MR, Gelesko S, Bell RB. Zygoma reconstruction. Oral Maxillofac Surg Clin North Am 2013; 25(2):167–201.

Management of Human and Animal Bites

James Murphy, DDS, MD[a], Mohammed Qaisi, DMD, MD[a,b],*

KEYWORDS

• Face • Animal bites • Human bites • Infection • Scarring • Cosmetics • Dog bite

KEY POINTS

- Dog bites are the most common facial animal bites.
- These wounds have a significant infection potential.
- The management includes not only surgical but also medical management.
- Management of animal and human bites is individualized based on each case.
- Dogs are the animal most frequently implicated in causing bite injuries to the human face.
- The oral flora of the animal that inflicts the bite or bites is a factor and has implications for management.
- Each species of animal has a relatively unique oral microbacterial flora, which has implications for the potential infection risk and the management of a wound.
- Bite wounds tend to result in 3 broad categories of injury: puncture wounds, lacerations, and tissue avulsion injuries.
- Dog bites tend to result in more lacerations and avulsive-type injuries.
- Cat bites tend to be more puncture-type wounds.
- Human bites to the face more commonly involve the ear, but the lip and nose also are sites with a higher incidence of human bite injury.

INTRODUCTION

The human face is a cosmetically and overly sensitive area, which is a critical component in our daily human interactions with others. Trauma to the facial tissues has immense social, psychological, and functional ramifications. Human and animal bites to the face tend to result predominantly in isolated soft tissue injury, but this soft tissue injury wound tends to be ragged and more prone to unfavorable scarring. The oral flora of the animal that inflicts the bite or bites is a factor and has implications for management. Most animal bites sustained by humans occur to the extremities, with less than 20% involving the face.[1] Dogs and to a lesser extent cats tend to be the most frequently involved animal in delivering the bite to humans in the developed world, but other animals, such as monkeys, horses, camels, bears, wild boars, rodents, sheep, pigs, snakes, fish, and crocodiles, have been documented in biting humans.[2] The importance of this is that each animal has a characteristic tooth shape and format that ultimately has an influence on the degree and type of injury. Each species of animal has a relatively unique oral microbacterial flora, which has implications for the potential infection risk and the management of a wound. Following dogs and cats, humans tend to be the third most common source of a bite injury to a fellow human. Unlike the above listed animals, a human bite has the potential to be used

The authors have no conflicts of interest to declare.
a Oral and Maxillofacial Surgery, Cook County Health, 1969 W. Ogden Avenue, Chicago, IL 60612, USA;
b Midwestern University, Chicago, IL, USA
* Corresponding author. Oral and Maxillofacial Surgery, Cook County Health, 1969 W. Ogden Avenue, Chicago, IL 60612.
E-mail address: moeqaisi@gmail.com

Oral Maxillofacial Surg Clin N Am 33 (2021) 373–380
https://doi.org/10.1016/j.coms.2021.04.006
1042-3699/21/© 2021 Elsevier Inc. All rights reserved.

to identify the aggressor based on forensic dentistry.

EPIDEMIOLOGY

With regards to public health, an estimated 2% of the population is bitten each year.[3] Animal bites are more prevalent in men and boys. With regards to cat and dog bites, there tends to be a sex predilection with regards to the human that sustains the bite injury. Women and girls are most likely to be bitten by cats, whereas men and boys tend to be bitten mostly by dogs. Dogs account for most facial bite wound injuries. The age of the human victim is also a factor to consider. Animal bites to the face are far more common in children than adults, with approximately 10% of bites involving the head and neck in adults compared with approximately 75% in children.[4] The reasoning behind this is that children tend to have less well-developed motor skills with which to defend themselves with their extremities. Children also tend to have larger heads with respect to their bodies, consequently making it a larger target. Last, children are less likely to be able to recognize the emotional behavior of animals, and as a result, do not appreciate the danger and may be more prone to provoking the animal.

WOUND CHARACTERISTICS AND CLASSIFICATION

Bite wounds tend to result in 3 broad categories of injury: puncture wounds, lacerations, and tissue avulsion injuries. Dog bites tend to result in more lacerations and avulsive-type injuries. Dog bite wounds are generally ragged and can have a component of crush injury. The breed of dog inflicting the injury also has an effect on the resulting wound. Pit bulls, terriers, and rottweilers tend to result in more ragged and avulsive injuries

because of their dental arrangement. These dogs also tend to have a more forceful bite, with some estimating the potential bite force to be up to 450 pounds per square inch.[5] A retrospective analysis of facial dog bites at a US trauma center showed bite wounds of some breeds of dogs were generally managed with direct repair, but other breeds, such as those noted above, tended to require reconstruction as part of the management of the dog bite injury.[6] This force is potentially strong enough to cause fractures of the human skeleton, especially in a child, and has the potential to cause death if inflicted on the skull. Dog bite injuries inflicted on the neck can be particularly serious, as airway damage with subsequent asphyxiation or great vessel injury with subsequent exsanguination is possible. Dog bites of the face tend to involve lips, nose, and cheek anatomic areas. Cat bites tend to be more puncture-type wounds. Cat bites tend to have a higher incidence of infection because of the penetrating nature of the injury and the microbiology of the cat oral cavity. Human bites to the face more commonly involve the ear, but the lip and nose also are sites with a higher incidence of human bite injury. To aid communication and to allow better assessment of outcomes with respect to varying facial bite wound injuries, Lackmann and colleagues[7] introduced a classification based on facial dog bit wound injuries in children, as shown in **Table 1**. The severity of bite wounds should be assessed, and a determination should be made if the bite wound is a high-risk bite wound. High-risk bite wounds generally require more urgent attention and have the potential to lead to significant complications. High-risk bite wounds include full-thickness puncture wounds, severe crush injury accompanying the bite injury, cat bite wounds, and bite wounds that involve bone, joint, tendon, and/or

Table 1	
Classification of facial bite wound injuries	
Type	**Clinical Findings**
I	Superficial injury without muscle involvement
IIA	Deep injury with muscle involvement
IIB	Full-thickness injury of the cheek or lip with oral mucosal involvement
IIIA	Deep injury with tissue defect
IIIB	Deep avulsive injury exposing nasal or auricular cartilage
IVA	Deep injury with severed facial nerve and/or parotid duct
IVB	Deep injury with concomitant bone fracture

ligament.[8] Facial bite wounds in of themselves are generally considered high risk without any of the above features though.

MICROBIOLOGY

The microbiology of animal bite wounds is polymicrobial. This polymicrobial wound environment is composed of a broad mixture of aerobic and anaerobic organisms. Commonly involved aerobic species include *Neisseria*, *Corynebacterium*, and *Staphylococcus*. Anaerobes most frequently implicated in animal bite wounds include *Fusobacterium*, *Bacteroides*, *Prevotella*, *Propionibacterium*, *Peptostreptococcus*, and *Porphyromonas*.

Focusing on the specifics of dog and cat bites, *Pasteurella* species, which is a gram-negative aerobic species and present in the oropharynx of most dogs and cats, is frequently implicated in dog and cat bite wound infections.[9] *Pasteurella canis* is found in 50% of dog bite wounds. *Pasteurella multocida* is found in approximately 30% of dog bite wounds and in approximately 50% of cat bite wounds. *Pasteurella* species bite wound infection can cause cellulitis in humans if not managed appropriately, and this can progress to purulent discharge, fever, osteomyelitis, septic arthritis, and ultimately, septicemia with its consequences if left unchecked.

Human bite wounds also tend to be polymicrobial. *Eikenella corrodens*, which is a normal commensal of the human oral cavity, appears to be particularly prevalent with respect to human bite wound infections. *Viridans streptococci* and *Streptococcus anginosus* tend to be relatively prevalent in human bite wound infections. In general, the aerobic and anaerobic organisms found in dog and cat bites tend to be otherwise similar in human bites with the exception of the *Pasteurella* species. A more worrisome point to consider with human bite injuries is the possibility of hepatitis B, hepatitis C, and HIV infection. These infections can be transferred from the human delivering the bite to the victim, especially if gingival trauma occurs to the person delivering the bite with resultant release of their blood, which can gain access to the victim. Consideration has to be given in human bite wound injuries for the potential of these microorganisms infecting the victim.

With animal bite wounds, the potential for rabies must be considered. Postexposure prophylaxis for rabies is essential and can prevent rabies in humans, which is currently untreatable. Postexposure prophylaxis consists of local wound treatment with washouts and cleaning of the wound followed by vaccination. Consideration should be given to the administration of rabies immune globulin dependingt on the type of exposure and the suspicion for being bitten by an animal suffering from rabies. The use of vaccination in conjunction with rabies immune globulin is essentially 100% effective in preventing human infection if inoculated by a bite from a rabies virus effected animal.

EVALUATION

Initial evaluation should focus on the principles of Advanced Trauma and Life Support (ATLS). Establishment of a defined airway and control of any hemorrhage are of particular importance and are relevant in pediatric patients. As part of the secondary survey, evaluation should be performed for any penetrating intracranial injuries that may result in a pediatric patient owing to their relatively less mineralized calvarial bones. Neurologic function should be assessed. With regards to the face, particular reference to facial nerve function and the sensory nerve function should also be evaluated and documented.

History and physical examination are of primary importance. As part of the history, documentation should be made of the timeline since the bite injury occurred. Ideally, patients with bite injuries to the face should be seen as soon as possible given that early management of the injury reduces the likelihood of infection. Bite injuries seen within 6 hours and managed appropriately have a lower risk of wound infection compared with those seen in a delayed fashion.[10] Animal bite wounds to the extremities are generally left open to reduce the risk of infection. With regards to the face, this is generally avoided to minimize the cosmetic impact of the injury. Bite wounds of the face seen and treated up to 48 hours after the injury with suturing have an acceptably low risk of infection but benefit from potential cosmetic benefits of suturing. There are advocates for suturing closed facial bite wounds presenting in a delayed fashion 48 hours or more after the injury.[11] On review of the patient's past medical history, one should pay particular attention to any conditions that may indicate an immunocompromised patient. Specific questions regarding the presence of diabetes, excessive alcohol consumption, a patient who is a transplant recipient, or a patient taking immunosuppressive drugs for autoimmune conditions should be elicited. The patient should be questioned on the use of tobacco with particular reference to smoking tobacco. This risk factor predisposes the patient to poor healing and an increased risk of infection.

As part of the clinical examination, any signs of infection should be documented, including but not limited to erythema, purulent drainage, or systemic signs of infection. With regards to the perioral and periorbital tissues, a clear description of the wound should be placed in the medical record. Any avulsed tissue should be noted with an accurately measured wound defect size obtained for the medical records. Medical photography can be invaluable in recording the injury. Injuries involving the perioral and periorbital tissues are high-risk injuries and put the patient at significant risk of cosmetic and functional impairment. Photodocumentation can also be very important in animal and human bite injuries, as these cases often have litigation consequences.

To aid proper assessment of the wound, any dried coagulation tissue or foreign body should ideally be removed with gentle saline irrigation. Excessive scrubbing should be avoided as part of the initial examination. To complete the examination, consideration should be given to radiological investigation. If there is any suspicion for fracture of the facial skeleton, strong consideration should be given to computed tomographic examination. If there is a concern for foreign body within the soft tissue, plain films may be suitable. Once a complete clinical, and if relevant, radiological examination, is completed, a discussion should be had with the patient with regards to their potential treatment options.

Surgical Management

All bite wound injuries should at least be irrigated with normal saline. There is minimal to no extra benefit in the addition of povidone iodine or hydrogen peroxide. Pulsed lavage also does not seem to be merited in most animal bite wound infections to the human face. Given the importance of facial cosmesis, facial bite wounds merit primarily closure with suturing if possible. In the process of primary closure, placement of deep sutures should be used judiciously, as these can act as a potential nidus for infection. A monofilament

nonabsorbable suture is preferable for skin reapproximation. The facial tissues have an abundant arterial supply; thus, minimal excision and debridement of tissue should be performed. If tissue is severely damaged and likely necrotic because of a crush injury or loss of vascularity, this should be removed, as it can act as a nidus for infection. An alternative strategy is minimal debridement and monitoring the wound with packing and repeated washouts and debridements until the treating provider is satisfied all necrotic material is removed before proceeding with closure/reconstruction of the wounds. Unfortunately, this management strategy is likely to have increased scarring, which ultimately is cosmetically detrimental.

Avulsive wounds with tissue loss require consideration for closure by secondary intention, local tissue rearrangement, skin grafting, or free tissue transfer depending on the size and the location of the defect. Cosmetically and functionally sensitive areas, such as the perioral tissues and periorbital tissues, require careful evaluation. Local rearrangement of tissue with advancement of mucosa and the skin of the lip may be sufficient to allow a cosmetic and functional result if orbicularis oris is intact (**Fig. 1**). With some avulsive lip injuries, consideration can be given to reimplanting the avulsed tissue if the patient is seen quickly following the injury (**Fig. 2**). This strategy is risky, and complete loss of the replaced avulsed tissue can occur frequently. Generally, if orbicularis oris is not intact, wedge resection with primary closure across the defect versus an Abbe or an Estlander flap may need to be considered (**Fig. 3**). Larger defects may require reconstruction with advancement flaps, like Fernandes, Bernard, or Karapandzic flaps. Complete loss of the lip will require free tissue transfer. With regards to the periorbital tissues, assessment of lacrimal system should be performed. Any defects in the lacrimal system require dacryocystorhinostomy. Reconstruction to allow functional return of the sphincter

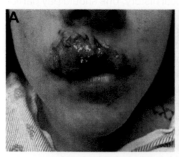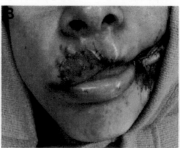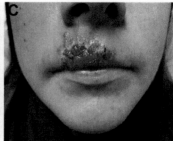

Fig. 1. Beagle dog bite to upper lip with loss of tissue. (*A*) Patient seen in the emergency department with dog bite to upper lip with loss of tissue. (*B*) Intraoperatively after washout and debridement with local tissue rearrangement. (*C*) Three weeks postoperatively with acceptable cosmesis.

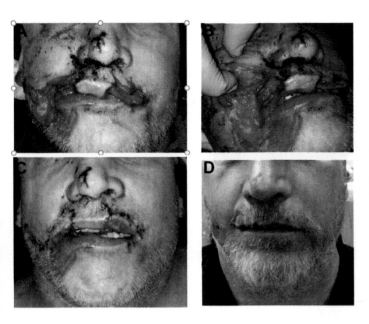

Fig. 2. Doberman dog bite with complete avulsion of the right upper lip. (*A*) Wound as seen in the emergency department approximately 2 hours after the injury. (*B*) Tissue reflected to show extent of tissue loss. Patient brought avulsed tissue. (*C*) Following washout and debridement with replacement of avulsed tissue right upper lip. (*D*) Three weeks postrepair. Vermillion survived. Some secondary healing in area of skin but relatively fair cosmetic result given extent of the injury.

mechanism of the periorbital and perioral tissues is of prime importance. Without return of the sphincter function, long-lasting and severe functional and cosmetic impediment will be the result.

Reconstruction of the nasal and ear defects can also be complex. Partial avulsions of the ear can

sometimes be reapproximated and reanastomosed without loss if a vascular pedicle is maintained. If this is performed, a bolster dressing needs to be placed. If partial avulsion occurs without maintenance of a vascular pedicle, either the pocket reconstruction method (**Fig. 4**) (Mladick

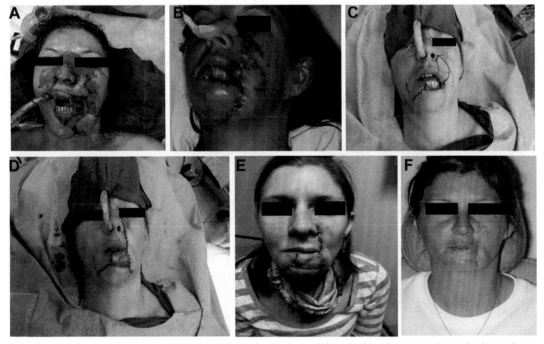

Fig. 3. (*A*) A 23-year-old woman with multiple facial lacerations and an avulsive injury involving the lower lip as a result of a dog bite by a pit bull. (*B*) After closure of lacerations primarily. (*C, D*) Delayed closure at 6 weeks with an Estlander flap. (*E*) One week postrepair. (*F*) Six weeks postrepair.

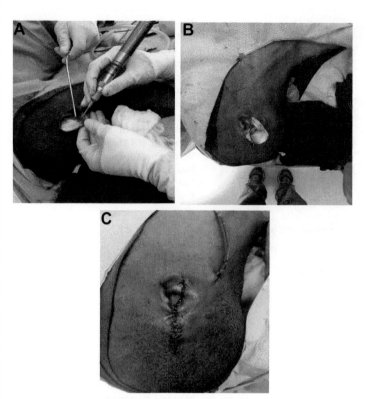

Fig. 4. Patient sustained a bite to his right ear during an altercation resulting in partial avulsion. (*A*) The avulsed portion sutured back primarily. (*B*) The avulsed portion deepithelialized with a diamond bur and (*C*) buried in a retroauricular pocket.

technique) or cartilage grafting with a temporoparietal fascia flap and skin flap can be used.[12] Complete avulsions of the ear may need either prosthetic replacement with an implant-retained prosthesis or complete reconstruction with rib cartilage grafting along with scalp skin flaps and temporoparietal fascia flap. With regards to the nose, soft tissue defects with maintenance of the underlying cartilage can be managed with either local tissue rearrangement or full-thickness skin grafting (**Fig. 5**). If a defect of the nasal cartilage occurs, cartilage grafting with pedicle flap or free tissue transfer may be required. Complete loss of nose may be managed with an implant-retained prosthesis by an anaplastologist. An osteocutaneous radial forearm free flap is also frequently used in total nasal defects.

With regards to animal bites affecting the area of the parotid gland, the treating provider needs to consider facial nerve damage and parotid duct

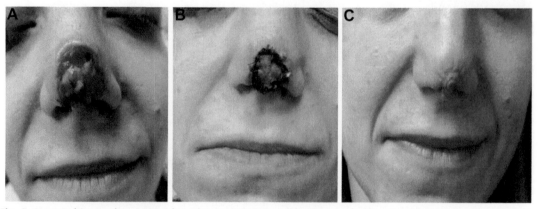

Fig. 5. Human bite to the nose with Lackmann IIIB injury. (*A*) One week after the injury with granulation in wound bed. (*B*) Two weeks after the injury with supraclavicular full-thickness graft 5 days in place. (*C*) Four weeks after the injury with full-thickness skin graft integrating well.

injuries. Injuries to the cheek on a line connecting the tragus of the ear to the upper lip where the philtrum meets the vermillion as defined by Van Sickels[13] should be viewed with suspicion for a parotid duct injury. To evaluate the parotid duct, a catheter can be inserted through Stensen duct intraorally and irrigated in a retrograde fashion. If irrigant is noted to be coming from the wound, then a parotid duct injury is present; this can be confirmed with sialography. Injury in the middle or distal portion of the parotid duct can be repaired. Injury of the parotid duct in the proximal third or within the gland is difficult to repair. Management of this type of parotid duct injury is best with Botox to the parotid gland, or pressure dressing with antisialagogues can be considered. If a sialocele develops, this can be managed with aspiration and sialagogues (**Fig. 6**). Injuries to the parotid duct signal possible injury to the buccal branch of the facial nerve because of their intimate relationship. If a facial nerve injury is suspected, the location of the facial nerve injury should be evaluated. Facial nerve injuries located distally along the branch are generally not repaired. As a rule of thumb, injuries to facial nerve branches at a point distal to a vertical dropped from the lateral canthus of the eye are not repaired. More proximal injuries on the facial nerve should ideally be explored within 72 hours of injury and repaired if possible. When repairing facial nerve injuries, no tension should be put on the repaired nerve, as this will increase the risk of failure. If any tension is present at reapproximation of the nerve, a nerve graft should be used. This scenario is often the case in traumatic injuries because of the edema of the surrounding tissues, which results in retraction of the severed nerve ends.

Animal bite injuries, and in particular dog bite injuries to the scalp, especially in pediatric patients, can result in significant hemorrhage. Hemorrhage

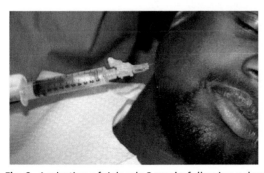

Fig. 6. Aspiration of sialocele 2 weeks following a dog bite to the right cheek with injury to intraglandular component of parotid duct.

control as part of the ATLS should already have been performed. When repairing an extensive scalp wound defect secondary to animal bites, consideration should be given to active draining suction placement. Active draining suction placement decreases the risk of this hematoma formation and subsequent infection with effective healing. Severe facial injuries with massive facial tissue loss can rarely occur following animal bites. The world's first successful face transplant was performed in 2005 in France on a 38-year-old female patient who sustained a facial dog bite with massive tissue loss.[14] The patient lost her lips, nose, and right periorbital tissues as a result of her injury. She underwent an allograft in 2005 in Amiens, France. The patient initially did well but, unfortunately, suffered from chronic rejection of the allograft and succumbed to malignancy because of her immunocompromised state and died in 2016. This case exemplifies not only that animal bite wounds to the face can be extremely disfiguring but also that patients are willing to undertake extreme and sometimes experimental therapies as part of their treatment.

Medical Management

Given the polymicrobial nature of animal bite wounds, antibiotic prophylaxis is strongly recommended. On the face, in the context of primary closure of the wound, the requirement for antibiotic prophylaxis is of the utmost importance in minimizing infection and subsequent sequelae of increased scarring and cosmetic impediment. Based on the previously discussed microbiology, amoxicillin/clavulanate is the antibiotic of choice. Amoxicillin/clavulanate has a good broad spectrum of activity and is active against most bacteria that are thought to be involved in dog, cat, and human bites. In a patient with allergy to penicillin, there is divergence of opinion with regards to the best alternative. Clindamycin is generally favored; however, in the authors' experience, clindamycin in isolation as a prophylactic antibiotic tends to have a relatively high risk of infection at the bite wound. If clindamycin is chosen, it should ideally be supplemented with either fluoroquinolone or trimethoprim sulfamethoxazole. Doxycycline is another alternative; however, its bacteriostatic effect it makes it less favorable than penicillin-based antibiotics. Moxifloxacin has good activity against most animal bite wound microbes with the exception of *Fusobacterium*. Its cost can sometimes be prohibitive. A macrolide like azithromycin is the least preferred empiric antibiotic to use in the treatment of animal bites. If a wound infection occurs, cultures should be obtained and submitted to microbiology to aid directed antimicrobial therapy. Consideration should be given to opening of the sutures and irrigating and debriding the wound.

The tetanus status of the patient should be ascertained. If the patient has not received a tetanus vaccine in 10 years, tetanus immunoglobulin with a tetanus vaccine should be administered. If a tetanus vaccine has not been delivered within 5 years, a tetanus vaccine should be administered and consideration given to tetanus immunoglobulin depending on the injury. As previously discussed, consideration should be also given to the possibility of rabies and the need for rabies postexposure prophylaxis. A special consideration for human bite wounds is the possibility of HIV, hepatitis B, and hepatitis C infection. Baseline blood tests should be drawn. Questions should be asked regarding the patient's history and exposure to HIV, hepatitis B, and hepatitis C, and this needs to be documented. Consideration should be given to postexposure prophylaxis for HIV. With regards to this, infectious disease expert should be involved.

Animal bites to the face in general tend to be very distressing psychological injuries. Consideration of the patient's coping mechanisms should be included in the evaluation and consideration for referral to psychiatry, which are particularly important with severe and disfiguring injuries.

SUMMARY

Animal bite wounds to the face can result in severe injuries that can have long-lasting consequences. Thankfully, most animal bite wounds to the face can be managed in an outpatient setting with close monitoring. Infection is always a risk but with modern understanding of the microbiology involved, relatively good empiric antibiotic therapy can be administered to reduce the risk of the consequences of infection. As most animal bite wounds to the face are caused by dogs, and most dog bite wounds of the face are in children, prevention should be a primary focus. Prevention can avoid not only the physical stress of the injury but also the inevitable psychological injury involved.

CLINICS CARE POINTS

- Dog and cat bites have a high incidence of Pasteurella infection.

- All animal bite wounds should be washed out.
- A penicillin-based antibiotic is preferable.
- Every attempt should be made to close facial bite wounds even with delayed presentation.

REFERENCES

1. Stefanopoulos PK. Management of facial bite wounds. Oral Maxillofac Surg Clin North Am 2009; 21:247–57.

2. Dendle C, Looke D. Management of mammalian bites. Aust Fam Physician 2009;38:868–74.

3. Dendle C, Looke D. Review article: animal bites: an update for management with a focus on infections. Emerg Med Australas 2008;20:458–67.

4. Chhabra S, Chhabra N, Gaba S. Maxillofacial injuries due to animal bites. J Maxillofac Oral Surg 2015;14:142–53.

5. Agrawal A, Kumar P, Singhal R, et al. Animal bite injuries in children: review of literature and case series. Int J Clin Pediatr Dent 2017;10:67–72.

6. Gurunluoglu R, Glasgow M, Arton J, et al. Retrospective analysis of facial dog bite injuries at a level I trauma center in the Denver metro area. J Trauma Acute Care Surg 2014;76:1294–300.

7. Lackmann GM, Draf W, Isselstein G, et al. Surgical treatment of facial dog bite injuries in children. J Craniomaxillofac Surg 1992;20:81–6.

8. Lewis KT, Stiles M. Management of cat and dog bites. Am Fam Physician 1995;52:479–85.

9. Talan DA, Citron DM, Abrahamian FM, et al. Bacteriologic analysis of infected dog and cat bites. Emergency Medicine Animal Bite Infection Study Group. N Engl J Med 1999;340:85–92.

10. Stefanopoulos PK, Tarantzopoulou AD. Management of facial bite wounds. Dent Clin North Am 2009;53:691–705.

11. Stefanopoulos PK, Tarantzopoulou AD. Facial bite wounds: management update. Int J Oral Maxillofac Surg 2005;34:464–72.

12. Maloney K. Partial avulsion of the right ear treated with a pocket technique: a case report and review of the literature. J Maxillofac Oral Surg 2015;14: 288–92.

13. Van Sickels JE. Parotid duct injuries. Oral Surg Oral Med Oral Pathol Oral Radiop Endod 1981;52:364–7.

14. Devauchelle B, Badet L, Lengelé B, et al. First human face allograft: early report. Lancet 2006;368: 203–9.

Management of Traumatic Trigeminal and Facial Nerve Injuries

Michael R. Markiewicz, DDS, MD, MPH[a,b,c,d,*],
Nicholas Callahan, MPH, DMD, MD[e,f], Michael Miloro, DMD, MD[e]

KEYWORDS

- Injuries • Trigeminal nerve • Facial nerve • Cranial nerve injury • Nerve graft • Nerve allograft
- Facial trauma • Maxillofacial trauma

KEY POINTS

- The inferior alveolar nerve, lingual nerve, infraorbital nerve, as well as other branches of the trigeminal nerve are at risk for injury as a result of craniomaxillofacial trauma.
- The facial nerve can be categorized into 3 distinct segments: the intracranial, intratemporal, and extratemporal segments.
- The Seddon classification, Sunderland classification, and Medical Research Council Scale are all ways to classify sensory nerve injuries.
- The House-Brackmann scale, or variants of this scale, is the preferred scale for evaluating and monitoring facial nerve injuries.

INTRODUCTION

Injury to the fifth (V, trigeminal) and seventh (VII, facial) cranial nerves may result in significant cosmetic and functional deficits. These deformities have a profound effect on quality of life. The head and neck region is rich in neural and vascular networks, and the density of peripheral nerve receptors in this area makes neurosensory disturbance more noticeable than in other parts of the body (eg, trunk and extremities). The trigeminal and facial nerves are the most common cranial nerves affected in maxillofacial trauma. Ultimately, the structures that they innervate are involved in nearly all cases of facial trauma. Unlike with other

mechanisms of injury, diagnosis of cranial nerve injury in maxillofacial trauma can be challenging because of the associated patient-oriented factors and the setting in which they are assessed. However, as in the nontrauma setting, expeditious management is critical to the best chance of neurosensory recovery. Injury to the trigeminal nerve can have a profound effect on speech and swallowing, taste, and mastication. Likewise, injury to the facial nerve may have deleterious effects on function and social interaction because it not only innervates the muscles of mastication but provides parasympathetic stimulation to the lacrimal, sublingual, and submandibular glands. This article reviews the diagnosis and

[a] Department of Oral and Maxillofacial Surgery, School of Dental Medicine, University at Buffalo, 3435 Main Street, 112 Squire Hall, Buffalo, NY 14214, USA; [b] Department of Neurosurgery, Jacobs School of Medicine and Biomedical Sciences, Buffalo, NY, USA; [c] Department of Neurosurgery, Division of Pediatric Surgery, Department of Surgery, Jacobs School of Medicine and Biomedical Sciences, Buffalo, NY, USA; [d] Craniofacial Center of Western New York, John Oishei Children's Hospital, Buffalo, NY, USA; [e] Department of Oral and Maxillofacial Surgery, University of Illinois at Chicago, Room 110, 801 S. Paulina Street, Chicago, IL 60612, USA; [f] Department of Otolaryngology, Northwestern Memorial Hospital, Chicago, IL, USA
* Corresponding author.
E-mail address: mrm25@buffalo.edu

Oral Maxillofacial Surg Clin N Am 33 (2021) 381–405
https://doi.org/10.1016/j.coms.2021.04.009
1042-3699/21/© 2021 Elsevier Inc. All rights reserved.

management of trigeminal and facial nerve injuries in the setting of craniomaxillofacial trauma. Standard use of terminology between clinicians is critical when managing peripheral nerve injuries. Commonly used to terms to describe neurosensory disturbances are listed in **Table 1**.

TRIGEMINAL NERVE
Macroanatomy

The trigeminal nerve is the largest of the cranial nerves. It has 3 divisions: the ophthalmic (V1), maxillary (V2), and mandibular (V3). The trigeminal nerve is unique in that it contains sensory (general afferent) and mixed motor (proprioceptive and special efferent) components. The third division of trigeminal nerve has 2 main branches: the inferior alveolar nerve (IAN) and the lingual nerve. This article does not discuss in detail injuries to the first division of the trigeminal nerve or other less commonly injured nerves, such as the buccal nerve or nerve to the mylohyoid muscle.

Inferior Alveolar Nerve

The mandibular division (V3) of the trigeminal nerve has 3 branches, with the IAN being the largest (**Fig. 1**). The third division of the trigeminal nerve exits the skull base through the foramen ovale of the greater wing of the sphenoid bone (see **Fig. 1**). It descends lateral to the medial pterygoid muscle and medial to the mandibular forearm. It enters the mandible through the mandibular foramen and then travels through the body of the mandible and exits the mental foramen. The IAN is most lateral and closest to the buccal cortex at the third molar region of the mandible. It then changes trajectory at the first molar region where it neighbors the lingual plate. At the area of the premolars, the IAN again travels adjacent to the buccal cortex before exiting the mental foramen.[1–3] Depending on race, the mental foramen may be located between the premolars (white people) or distal to the second molar (black people).[4] The superior extent of the lingual nerve is at the lingula, 100 mm from the sigmoid notch. It reaches its most caudal aspect at the region between the first molar and second premolar. At this landmark, its splits into the incisive and mental nerve branches and it is 7.5 mm ($\pm$1 mm) from the inferior border of the mandible. The IAN provides sensory innervation to the mandibular teeth.

The mental nerve is a continuation of the IAN as it exits the mental foramen (see **Fig. 1**) and is frequently at risk for injury with parasymphysis and body fractures of the mandible. It has 2 main branches; however, up to 4 subdivisions can be seen (angular, medial inferior labial, lateral inferior labial, and mental).[5] The orbicularis oris branch, the largest branch, runs just beneath the mucosa and superficial to the orbicularis oris muscle. This branch can easily be injured on a transoral approach to the mandibular body or symphysis. Care should be taken to dissect this nerve during the approach to the mandible (see **Fig. 1**). The labial branch innervates the mucosa of the lip and chin. Another smaller mucosal branch travels posteriorly to innervate the buccinator muscle.

Lingual Nerve

The lingual nerve emanates from the posterior division of the third division of the trigeminal nerve. It travels medial to the lateral pterygoid muscle on a course medial to the IAN (see **Fig. 1**A). It then travels between the ramus and medial pterygoid muscle within mesioneural fat. The lingual nerve then enters the oral cavity as it travels over the

Table 1	
Select terminology of sensory alterations	
Term	**Definition**
Allodynia	Pain because of a nonpainful stimulus
Analgesia	Absence of pain from a painful stimulation
Anesthesia	Absence of any sensation from a painful or nonpainful stimulation
Dysesthesia	Abnormal sensation, spontaneous or evoked, that is unpleasant
Hyperalgesia	Abnormal response to a painful stimulus
Hyperesthesia	Increased sensitivity to stimulation, excludes special senses
Hyperpathia	Increased reaction to a (repetitive) stimulus
Hypoalgesia	Diminished pain in response to a painful stimulus
Hypoesthesia	Decreased sensitivity to stimulation; excludes special senses
Neuralgia	Pain in the distribution of a nerve or nerves
Paresthesia	An abnormal sensation, spontaneous or evoked, that is not unpleasant

From Schlieve T, Miloro M, and Kolokythas A. Chapter 5: Diagnosis and Management of Trigeminal and Facial Nerve Injuries. In: Fonseca, R, ed. Oral and Maxillofacial Surgery. 3rd ed. 2018: 70-113; with permission.

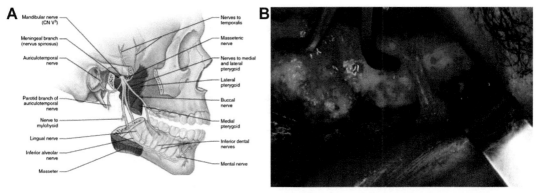

Fig. 1. (*A*) Regional anatomy showing the peripheral trigeminal nerve system. (*B*) View of the mental nerve as it exits the mental foramen. (*From* Miloro M, Kolokytas A. Chapter 25: Traumatic Injuries of the Trigeminal Nerve. In: Fonseca, R, ed. Oral and Maxillofacial Trauma. 4th ed. Elsevier; 2012: 650-682; with permission.)

superior pharyngeal constrictor, styloglossus, and mylohyoid muscles. The nerve then travels from lateral to medial at the level of the third molar position. It provides sensory and special sensory function to the anterior two-thirds of the ipsilateral tongue, floor of mouth, and lingual mandibular gingiva. The lingual nerve merges with the chorda tympani branch of the facial nerve as it travels through the petrotympanic fissure. This nerve provides taste to the anterior two-thirds of the tongue and carries special visceral afferents, including preganglionic parasympathetic fibers to the submandibular and sublingual glands. At the level of the sigmoid notch there are 4 branching patterns of the IAN and lingual nerve[6]: separation above the sigmoid notch and inferior to the otic ganglion (65.6%), separation below the notch and at the superior half of the distance between the notch and ganglia (28%), separation below the notch and at the inferior half of the distance between the notch and lingula (3.1%), and separation in a plexiform pattern (6.3%). The bifurcation occurs at a mean distance of 14.3 mm (7.8–24.1 mm) inferior to the foramen ovale and 16.5 mm superior to the tipoff the hamulus (4.9–24.3 mm). There are collateral branches to the retromolar trigone in 81% of cases owing to the commonly reported failure rate of mandibular anesthesia.[6]

In the area of the third molar, the lingual nerve can be found superior to the lingual crest in 10% of people, and in direct contact with the lingual plate in 25%.[7] At the third molar region, the lingual nerve has a diameter between 2 and 5 mm. The shape varies between being round, oval, kidney shaped, elliptical, or ribbonlike in cross section; however, the predominant shape varies between studies.[6–14] The exact location of the lingual nerve in the third molar region varies between studies (**Table 2**). When adjacent to the second molar, the lingual nerve crosses the Wharton duct from lateral to medial traveling below the duct and hypoglossal nerve in the submandibular triangle. In this region, that the lingual nerve gives off preganglionic parasympathetic fibers from the facial nerve to the submandibular ganglion. The lingual nerve may be damaged on excision of the submandibular gland in up to 1.4% to 4.8% of patients.[15] After looping under the Wharton duct, the lingual nerve travels cephalad and enters the genioglossus muscle and tongue substance. One to 2 branches travel to the tip of the tongue. Other branches travel to the lingual mucosa and gingiva and are of small diameter (1–2 mm).[16]

Infraorbital Nerve

The infraorbital nerve (ION) is a terminal branch of the second division of the trigeminal nerve and becomes extracranial at the foramen rotundum. It emerges through the skeleton onto the face at the infraorbital foramen. The mean distance of the infraorbital foramen from the facial midline and inferior orbital rim is 2.7 cm and 6 to 8 mm respectively.[16,17] There is usually 1 canal (90%), with 2 canals (5%) or 3 canals being present (5%) in fewer cases. The shape of the canal may be oval (30%), round (40%), or semilunar (30%).[17] The infraorbital nerve exits the infraorbital foramen to divide into 4 branches, supplying the midface, nose, upper lip, and lower eyelid.[18]

The ION enters the orbit via the inferior orbital fissure and travels posteriorly. The canal may not be complete, and a groove rather than a canal is seen in 50% of cases. The ION is at risk during periorbital approaches and during fractures involving the midface or neighboring structures.

MICROANATOMY

The microanatomy of all peripheral nerves, sensory or motor, is similar, with a ratio of myelinated

Table 2
Distances and relationship of lingual nerve to mandible at third molar region

Study	Nerves (N)	Vertical Measurement (mm)	Horizontal Measurement (mm)	Lingual Nerve Above Alveolar Crest (%)	Lingual Nerve in Contact With Lingual Plate (%)
Kiesselbach & Chamberlain,[8] 1984	34 cadaveric and 256 in vivo nerves	2.28 ± 1.96	0.58 ± 0.9	17.6	62
Pogrel et al,[14] 1995	40 cadaveric nerves	8.32 ± 4.05	3.45 ± 1.48	15	0
Behnia et al,[13] 2000	669 cadaveric nerves	3.01 ± 0.42	2.06 ± 1.10	14.05	23.27
Holzle & Wollfe,[12] 2011	68 cadaveric nerves	7.83 ± 1.65	0.86 ± 1.00	8.82	57.4
Karakas et al,[11] 2007	21 cadaveric nerves	9.56 ± 5.28	4.19 ± 1.99	4.7	0
Miloro et al,[7] 1997	20 in vivo nerves (evaluated by high-resolution MRI)	2.75 ± 1.00	2.53 ± 0.67	10	25

From Schlieve T, Miloro M, and Kolokythas A. Chapter 5: Diagnosis and Management of Trigeminal and Facial Nerve Injuries. In: Fonseca, R, ed. Oral and Maxillofacial Surgery. 3rd ed. 2018: 70-113; with permission.

to unmyelinated fibers of 1:4. Sensory and motor peripheral nerves differ in the number of Schwann cells surrounding each fiber with nodes of Ranvier that permit saltatory nerve conduction (**Fig. 2**).The membrane, or basal lamina, created by the Schwann cell wraps around the axon and runs the entire length of the axon. This structure is often called the band of bungner (laminar myelin sheath) and is crucial in the process of nerve regeneration. Although myelin may be destroyed during injury, the Schwann cells often survive. This process plays a supportive role in nerve repair and regeneration. The internode is the length of axon surrounded by a single Schwann cell. The small area (0.3 μm to 2.0 μm) between the internodes where the axon is not myelinated is known as the node of Ranvier. The nodes of Ranvier allow the diffusion of certain ions, causing nerve depolarization and repolarization. This process allows conduction of nerve impulses along the nerve fiber. It is this conduction between nodes of Ranvier (saltatory conduction) that is responsible for the rapid transmission of nerve impulses in myelinated nerves (up to 150 m/s) compared with nonmyelinated nerve fibers (2–2.5 msec).

In general, unmyelinated axons are smaller in diameter than myelinated nerves (0.15–2.0 μm). Collagen creates the surrounding framework of the nerve and contributes to the structural architecture of the nerve. The endoneurium is the collagen covering surrounding each nerve fiber axon (**Fig. 3**).[19,20] Several of endoneurial groups, which are known as fascicles, are grouped together and surrounded by a second layer of collagen cells known as perineurium. The outermost layer supporting the nerve along with some elastic fibers is known as the epineurium (extrafascicular epineurium). The internal epineurium is another layer of epineurium that invests the fascicles. The epineurium consists of 50% of the cross-sectional area of the nerve. It provides a layer of protection again compression and other types of trauma. The final and outermost layer of the nerve, containing connective tissue and continuous with the epineurium and surrounding tissue, is the mesoneurium, or adventitia of the nerve.[19]

Peripheral nerves are often classified based on their fascicular pattern, including monofascicular, oligofascicular, and polyfascicular. Monofascicular nerves, such as the chorda tympani, have only 1 large fascicle. Oligofascicular nerves, such as the labial branch of the mental nerve, contain 2 to 10 fascicles. Polyfascicular nerves, such as inferior alveolar or lingual nerves, contain more than 10 fascicles. As cranial nerves travel from proximal to distal, in general the number of fascicles and cross-sectional area decrease.[21–23] **Table 3** reports the number of fascicles and diameter of common branches of the trigeminal nerve.

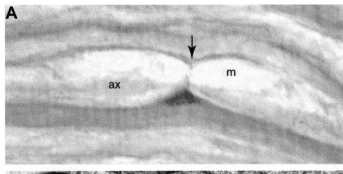

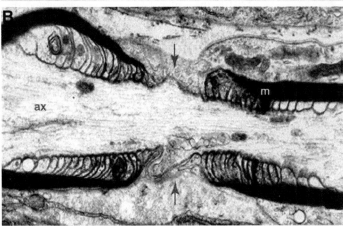

Fig. 2. Hematoxylin-eosin (*A*) and silver (*B*) stains showing the organization of a peripheral myelinated nerve in longitudinal section in the area of a node of Ranvier (*arrows*). ax, axon; m, myelin. (*From* Miloro M, Kolokytas A. Chapter 25: Traumatic Injuries of the Trigeminal Nerve. In: Fonseca, R, ed. Oral and Maxillofacial Trauma. 4th ed. Elsevier; 2013: 650-682; with permission.)

The blood supply of a nerve is usually provided by an associated artery and vein. Nerve fascicles have their own independent blood supplies, which is similar to individual nerve fibers (**Fig. 4**).[24,25] The vasculature passes between the layers of connective tissue within the intrafascicular layers. The vessels travel to the extrafascicular epineurium via the vasa nervosum, running in a longitudinally oriented plexus.

Epidemiology

Inevitably, all structures innervated by cranial nerves V and VII are involved in patients with oral and maxillofacial trauma. The structures that develop from the first and second branchial arches receive their innervation via the second and third divisions of the trigeminal nerve and facial nerve respectively. Therefore, the second and, more commonly, third divisions of the trigeminal nerve and any branch of the facial nerve may be damaged when trauma involves nearby structures. The facial nerve is affected in 48% of ballistic injuries to the temporal bone. Transection of the facial nerve may occur when tethered in the temporal bone or by tearing or crushing the nerve on exiting the temporal bone.

Diagnosis

Trigeminal nerve imaging

Radiologic examination of the trigeminal nerve for injury should be guided by clinical examination. Imaging of cranial nerves, especially that their distal aspects, has not made the same progress in recent decades as imaging of other bodily structures. Imaging of the trigeminal nerve should be categorized with regard to timing[26] (more specifically, the preinjury, postinjury, and postrepair phases). A fourth phase of intraoperative monitoring may be used as well (ie, witnessing a nerve injury or monitoring nerve conduction). The postinjury phase can be divided into the primary phase (immediately after injury) and secondary phase (ie, after nerve injury and repair).

Preoperative phase In the trauma setting, the preoperative assessment of the trigeminal nerve can only be done by obtaining imaging taken before nerve injury. Often this is not available. However, the surgeon should make attempts to acquire imaging (plain films, computed tomography [CT], MRI, and so forth). Evaluation of the preinjury status in the trigeminal nerve can include a panoramic radiograph, and plain films or CT scans of the head, face, and neck. Any disruption seen in the

A

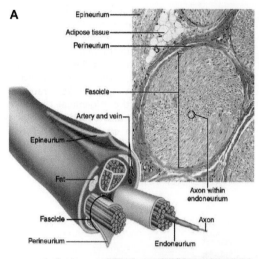

B

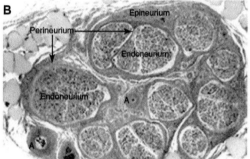

Fig. 3. (*A*) Nerve organization. (*B*) Low-power cross section of polyfascicular nerve showing the organization of the nerve, with individual nerve fibers surrounded by perineurium, and the investing epineurium. The mesoneurium is visible surrounding the entire nerve sheath at the periphery, with adipose tissue (*upper left*). A, perineurial and endoneurial blood vessels. (*From* Miloro M, Kolokytas A. Chapter 25: Traumatic Injuries of the Trigeminal Nerve. In: Fonseca, R, ed. Oral and Maxillofacial Trauma. 4th ed. Elsevier; 2013: 650-682; with permission.)

postinjury phase, not present on the preinjury panoramic radiograph, can help guide the surgeon to an area of needed exploration and possible repair.

CT bone windows are useful for assessing disruption of the cortical pathway of any neural canal, including the IAN canal. However, bone windows of CT are poor at visualizing neurovascular strictures and therefore cannot give any information about the structural integrity of the nerve itself. Soft tissue windows also give poor resolution for viewing neurovascular structures. In addition, dental artifacts, often present on CT scans of the head and neck, can make visualization of soft tissue structures challenging. Cone beam CT (CBCT) technology is an alternative to traditional CT for imaging of maxillofacial structures, but does not offer any additional detail compared with traditional CT, and it may offer less reliable data for neurovascular structures. Although both CBCT and CT can offer excellent visualization of the inferior alveolar canal or infraorbital foramen, both entities are poor at visualizing nerves contained within soft tissues, such as the lingual nerve or buccal nerve. If possible, CBCT should be used as an alternative to CT because it follows the rule: as low as reasonably achievable.

MRI is the optimal imaging for visualizing the nerve itself. Each segment of the nerve and the surrounding soft tissue structures around the nerve can be visualized in detail with MRI. Various settings, including coil selection, in-plane resolution, and use of other techniques, can be specified for visualization of the cranial nerves. Contrast-enhanced T1-weighted (T1W) or T1W three-dimensional fast filled echo imaging can be used to trace the third division of the trigeminal nerve as it exits the foramen ovale. It can then be traced further as it divides into the inferior alveolar and lingual nerves.[27–31] MRI is rarely available to identify cranial nerves in the preoperative setting. Mostly it is used to identify disorder or injury.[32–35] Ultrasonography is mainly used to assess peripheral nerve lesions. Although the advantage of ultrasonography is that it is readily available and inexpensive, because of the conspicuous nature, its use to assess the trigeminal nerve is limited.

Postinjury phase Panoramic radiograph is critical in assessing the postinjury phase in injuries to the lingual nerve and IAN. Cortical disruption and radiopaque foreign bodies can often be seen. Gross disruption of the inferior alveolar canal in the setting of mandible fracture may show an area of disruption and predict neurosensory changes.

Postinjury CT or CBCT may provide a more precise location of injury than panoramic radiography. Disruption along any aspect of the bony inferior alveolar nerve canal can be seen and indicates IAN injury. Disruption of the lingual cortex of the mandible in the third molar region caused by traumatic bony encroachment, or the presence of foreign bodies, along the perceived path of the lingual nerve may indicate injury.

Magnetic source imaging (MSI) is an entity that combines magnetoencephalography (MEG) and high-resolution MRI (HR-MRI). MEG works similarly to somatosensory evoked potentials, where a peripheral stimulus is applied and a central signal is recorded. This technique allows the measurement of both latency and amplitude of response. This information is then combined with HR-MRI

Table 3
Number of fascicles and diameter of branches of trigeminal nerve

Nerve	No. of Fascicles (Mean)	Mean Cross-sectional Area (mm²)
IAN	9.4–21 ± 7.05 (third molar region)	1.64 ± 0.27 (third molar region)
LN	8.5–10 ± 4.0 (third molar region)	1.87 ± 0.38 (third molar region)
MN	10.9–12 ± 3.58	1.18 ± 0.27
ION	5–6 (in the IOC)	2 (in the IOC) 0.4 (after it exits the IOF)

Abbreviations: IOC, infraorbital canal; IOF, infraorbital foramen; LN, lingual nerve; MN, mandibular nerve.

From Miloro M, Kolokytas A. Chapter 25: Traumatic Injuries of the Trigeminal Nerve. In: Fonseca, R, ed. Oral and Maxillofacial Trauma. 4th ed. Elsevier; 2013: 650-682; with permission.

to produce a functional and structural source image (MSI) of a region of the brain. MSI has been shown to differentiate different grades of IAN injury.[36]

HR-MRI is still a technology in its infancy. HR-MRI can possibly be used to identify prognosis of neurosensory return in patients with nerve injury caused by trauma.[37] HR-MRI also provides a more precise view of change in nerve position, including retraction of the nerve and neuroma formation in the area of injury. HR-MRI may also be able to show a change in nerve shape, which can lead to the diagnosis of neuroma formation.[38] HR-MRI may also be useful in monitoring the progression of anatomic neurosensory recovery following nerve injury and/or microneurosurgical repair, and this is an area of further study.[26]

Perhaps the most exciting imaging modality to assess nerve injury is magnetic resonance neurography (MRN). Similar to magnetic resonance angiography, which focuses the application of MRI

technology to the blood vessels, MRN is direct imaging of neural structures. MRN images are obtained using axial, coronal, and longitudinal T_1 and T_2 image acquisition with customized phased array coils and imaging protocols. MRN is unique in that it can differentiate between surrounding soft tissue structures such as blood vessels, adipose tissue, and lymph nodes. Most research on MRN has focused on large peripheral nerves.[33,39–43] MRN can detect increased diameter of injured nerves, increase signal intensity, and longitudinal variations associated with nerve injury and recovery. Hyperintensity on MRN has not been correlated with degree of nerve injury. Signal hyperintensity has been shown after neurorrhaphy. MRN can depict fascicular architecture based on a difference in fluid composition of the neural elements. The advantage of MRN compared with other imaging techniques is that it is able to correlate imaging findings with histologic characteristics of different grades of nerve injuries as classified by Seddon and Sunderland.

CLASSIFICATION OF TRIGEMINAL INJURIES

The 2 most common nerve injury classification schemes are the Seddon and Sunderland. The Seddon classification is based on time between injury and recovery and degree of recovery. Sunderland emphasizes specific histologic degree or damaged neural structures.

Seddon Classification

The Seddon classification is a simple system that classifies nerve injuries into 3 levels of injury (**Fig. 5**): neurapraxia, axonotmesis, and neurotmesis. The integrity of the axon is maintained in neuropraxic injuries. In these types of injuries, there is a local conduction block from a transient anoxic event caused by acute disruption of the epineurial or endoneurial vasculature. Neurapraxia is often a result of minor nerve manipulation, compression, or traction injury. This condition is characterized

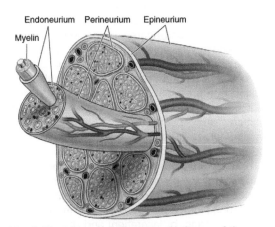

Endoneurium Perineurium Epineurium
Myelin

Fig. 4. Vascular supply between the layers of the connective tissue surrounding the axon (*red*, arteries; *blue*, veins). (*From* Miloro M, Kolokytas A. Chapter 25: Traumatic Injuries of the Trigeminal Nerve. In: Fonseca, R, ed. Oral and Maxillofacial Trauma. 4th ed. Elsevier; 2013: 650-682; with permission.)

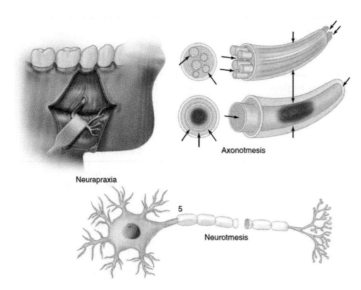

Neurapraxia

Axonotmesis

5

Neurotmesis

Fig. 5. Seddon classification system, including examples of neurapraxia, with nerve stretching, axonotmesis, with variable degrees of axonal injury, and neurotmesis, with nerve transection. (*From* Miloro M, Kolokytas A. Chapter 25: Traumatic Injuries of the Trigeminal Nerve. In: Fonseca, R, ed. Oral and Maxillofacial Trauma. 4th ed. Elsevier; 2013: 650-682; with permission.)

by a reversible conduction block with a favorable outcome with rapid and complete recovery within a few weeks of onset. There is no axonal degeneration in neuropraxic injuries, with damaged confined to the endoneurium only. However, axonotmesis is characterized by axonal damage and corresponds to Sunderland II to IV injuries. There is a variable degree of demyelination and axonal injury, which is why spontaneous recovery varies by category of injury. Neurotmesis is near-compete or complete transection with epineural discontinuity. Spontaneous recovery is unlikely and neuroma formation may occur.

Sunderland Classification

In 1951, Sunderland[44] revised and further subclassified nerve injuries into a 5-tiered system (**Table 4**). This system was based on histologic findings and degree of nerve involvement (**Fig. 6**).[44] A first-degree Sunderland injury is similar to Seddon neuropraxia. This classification was further divided by Sunderland into 3 types based on the severity and recovery time. A first-degree type 1 injury is the result of nerve manipulation that causes transient blood supply interruption. Once this is restored, it allows full sensory recovery after only a few hours. A first-degree type II injury involves intrafascicular edema formation from exudate or transudate. This condition usually results from moderate traction or compression injury to the nerve. Neurosensory recovery occurs after the edema resolves in the first few days. First-degree type III is characterized by intrafascicular edema formation resulting from transudate and exudate and results from moderate

traction, or compression on the nerve. Recovery of sensation is usually correlated with resolution of edema (several days after injury). First-degree type III injury results from even more aggressive nerve manipulation. Segmental demyelination may be present and recovery often takes a few days to weeks.[45] Second-degree injuries involve axonal and myelin interruption but intact endoneurium, epineurium, and perineurium, which allows axonal regeneration. Recovery may be slow and takes up to 1 year for complete return of normal sensation. Intact supporting and connective tissue structures may play an important role. Second-degree injuries are caused by traction or compression of the nerve. Third-degree injuries involve the endoneurium, whereas the epineurium and perineurium remain intact. Cause is similar to first-degree and second-degree injury, and spontaneous recovery is expected. However, complete recovery is not likely. Surgical exploration should be considered. Fourth-degree injuries result from traction, compression, needle injection, or chemical injury and can lead to disruption of the endoneurium and perineurium. The epineurium remains intact. Fourth-degree injuries have a poor potential or spontaneous recovery and a high probability of neuroma formation and intraneural fibrosis. Surgical intervention is required for these injuries. A fifth-degree Sunderland injury corresponds to Seddon's neurotmesis (nerve transection, avulsion, or laceration) and disruption of all components of the nerve. There is very little chance of spontaneous recovery. Extensive fibrous changes, neuroma formation, and neuropathic changes are seen. Spontaneous recovery

Table 4
Classification of nerve injuries and associated findings

Injury Type	Histologic Findings	Response	Recovery Pattern	Recovery Rate	Treatment
First degree (Seddon neuropraxia)	Transient ischemia, anoxia, ± segmental demyelination, intrafascicular edema	Conduction block	Complete	Fast (hours to weeks)	None indicated
Second degree (Seddon axonotmesis)	Axon and myelin interruption, (intact endoneurium, perineurium, and epineurium)	Wallerian degeneration distal to injury	Complete	Slow (weeks)	None indicated
Third degree	Injury involves endoneurium (intact perineurium and epineurium)	Wallerian degeneration and some degree of neuron cell death	Variable	Slow (weeks to months)	Nerve exploration may be considered
Fourth degree	Injury involves endoneurium and perineurium	Wallerian degeneration, neuron cell death, neuroma formation, intrafascicular fibrosis	None	Spontaneous recovery not likely	Microneurosurgery
Fifth degree (Seddon neurotmesis)	Complete nerve transection, continuity disruption	Wallerian degeneration, cell death, neuroma, fibrosis	None	No spontaneous recovery possible	Microneurosurgery

From Miloro M, Kolokytas A. Chapter 25: Traumatic Injuries of the Trigeminal Nerve. In: Fonseca, R, ed. Oral and Maxillofacial Trauma. 4th ed. Elsevier; 2013: 650-682; with permission.

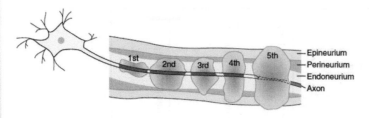

Fig. 6. Sunderland classification system showing the 5 degrees of nerve injury with progressive injury beginning with damage confined with the endoneurium (first-degree injury) and extending outward to the perineurium (second degree), then through the perineurium (third degree), and to the epineurium (fourth degree), and finally through the epineurium with discontinuity (fifth degree). (*From* Miloro M, Kolokytas A. Chapter 25: Traumatic Injuries of the Trigeminal Nerve. In: Fonseca, R, ed. Oral and Maxillofacial Trauma. 4th ed. Elsevier; 2013: 650-682; with permission.)

is very rare, and microsurgical repair is indicated when able. In the case of witnessed nerve transection, immediate surgical intervention is advocated.

Medical Research Council Scale

The Medical Research Council Scale is a nerve injury scale used to grade peripheral nerve injuries (**Table 5**).[46–48] The scale is graded S0 to S4. S0 is the absence of sensation, S1 is presence of deep cutaneous pain, S2 is recovery of superficial cutaneous pain and some tactile sensation, S3 is return

Table 5
Classification of sensory recovery (Medical Research Council system)

Grade (Stage)	Recovery of Sensibility
S0	No recovery
S1	Recovery of deep cutaneous pain
S1+	Recovery of some superficial pain
S2	Return of some superficial pain and tactile sensation
S2+	S2 with over-response
S3[a]	Return of some superficial pain and tactile sensation without over-response; 2-point discrimination >15 mm
S3+	S3 with good stimulus localization; 2-point discrimination = 7–15 mm
S4	Complete recovery; S3+; 2-point discrimination = 2–6 mm

[a] S3 indicates important clinical recovery.

Adapted from Wyrick JD, Stern PJ. Secondary nerve reconstruction. Hand Clin. 1992 Aug;8(3):587-98 and Mackinnon SE. Surgical management of the peripheral nerve gap. Clin Plast Surg. 1989 Jul;16(3):587-603; with permission.

of superficial cutaneous pain and tactile sensibility without over-response, and S4 is complete recovery. The drawback of this scale is that it is based on subjective findings and vague, nonstandardized data.

BIOLOGICAL RESPONSE TO INJURY

In general, nerve injury and repair follow the same set of postinjury events and reparative processes as other tissues.[49,50] After injury, the changes that occur within the cell body and nerve fiber depend on the proximity of the injury to the cell body as well as the severity of injury. Within 6 hours of injury, the metabolic rate of the cell body significantly increases, resulting in edema and migration of the nucleus toward the periphery of the cell body. There is an upregulation of the tough endoplasmic reticulum (Nissl substance), with increased protein synthesis that is exported from the cell body to the site of injury. These described events, known as chromatolysis, represent a histologic correlation of RNA and protein synthesis, a programmed event that is intended to ensure cell survival that peaks within 14 to 21 days of the injury.[51–59] In injuries that involve the axonal fibers (Sunderland II–V grade injuries) a series of events known as wallerian degeneration occurs throughout the distal nerve trunk and a minute portion of the proximal end close to the injury.[60] The distal end of the nerve becomes edematous and its ends are sealed. The myelin surrounding the axon breaks down into droplets and is phagocytosed by Schwann cells, which show enhanced proliferation and activity, and macrophages are recruited to the site.[61] These events are in preparation for attempted nerve regeneration and are completed within 1 week following nerve injury.[62–65] The final result is empty endoneurial tubes that act as conduits during nerve regeneration.[66–68] Proximally transected axons form sprouts that mimic axon growth cones observed during embryonic neural development. This highly productive activity of the Schwann cells is required for productions of new myelin that will host new axons. When these processes are interrupted or take place in an unusual order, neuroma formation may occur. Neuromas may be asymptomatic or symptomatic, and are sometimes painful (**Fig. 7**). Although clear transection injuries can be repaired primarily, avulsive injuries should be repaired in a delayed fashion roughly 3 weeks after the injury to allow for the extent of the injury to be well delineated. In addition, at this time neurotropic factors are at their highest levels and most supportive of repair.

MECHANISM OF INJURY TO THE TRIGEMINAL NERVE

Common causes of trigeminal nerve injury include local anesthetic injection, third molar surgery, dental implant surgery, orthognathic surgery, maxillofacial disorder, endodontic therapy, and chemical injury. However, trigeminal nerve injury in relation to trauma is discussed later.

Maxillofacial Trauma

Although it varies in the literature, the overall incidence of neurosensory disturbance of the trigeminal nerve in maxillofacial trauma is 71%, and, in the case of nondisplaced fractures, 88%.[69]

Cranial Nerve V: Second Division

Posttraumatic neurosensory disturbance of the infraorbital nerve occurs in more than 52% of midface fracture and zygomaticomaxillary complex (ZMC) fractures.[70] The infraorbital nerve, which is a terminal branch of the maxillary nerve, travels through the infraorbital fissure, through the infraorbital canal, and exits though the infraorbital foramen. It provides sensation to the entire cheek, upper lip, and ala of the nose.[71] Patients with blunt trauma to the midface with or without Le Fort or ZMC fractures may experience neurosensory disturbance to the infraorbital nerve (upper lip, cheek, perialar region). In addition to its other 4 articulations (sphenozygomatic, frontozygomatic, zygomaticomaxillary, and zygomaticotemporal sutures), ZMC fractures often propagate through

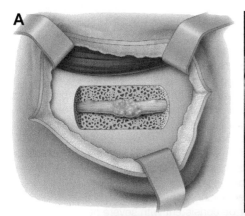
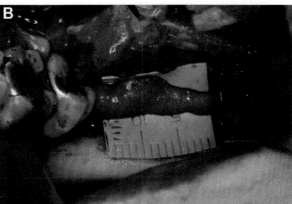
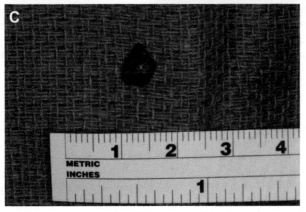

Fig. 7. (*A*) A fusiform neuroma in continuity. (*B*) Neuroma of the lingual nerve after exposure. (*C*) Neuroma specimen excised. ([*A*] *Adapted from* Miloro M, Kolokytas A. Chapter 25: Traumatic Injuries of the Trigeminal Nerve. In: Fonseca, R, ed. Oral and Maxillofacial Trauma. 4th ed. Elsevier; 2013: 650-682; with permission.)

the infraorbital fissure and infraorbital canal, lending to the name zygomatic-orbital-maxillary complex fracture.[72] Other causes of injury to the infraorbital nerve include ballistic injury, or penetrating wounds. In the setting of complete or partial neurosensory disturbance from nerve compression caused by facial fracture or blunt trauma and associated soft tissue edema, patients can expect partial to full recovery without intervention. Although neurosensory disturbance of the infraorbital nerve occurs in 65% of midface fractures, this only persists 15% of the time following treatment.[70] However, in the setting of witnessed transection of the infraorbital nerve either by examination after penetrating injury or after exposure during fracture repair, formal repair is advocated.

Cranial Nerve V: Third Division, Inferior Alveolar Nerve

Posttraumatic neurosensory disturbance of the IAN occurs in 56% to 76.9% of mandible fractures.[70,73,74] Neurosensory recovery is delayed in the setting of displaced fractures compared with nondisplaced fractures.[70,73] Neurosensory disturbance in the distribution of the IAN has been found to persist in 46% of patients 1 year following treatment. One study showed that, in 66.7% of patients with posttreatment neurosensory disturbance, the deficit was permanent.[73] Compression injuries of the IAN may result in the most significant neurosensory deficits.[75]

CLINICAL NEUROSENSORY TESTING

Neurosensory testing (NST) should be performed for patients with neurosensory changes to determine the degree of sensory impairment, monitor recovery, and to assist with clinical decision making and the need for surgical intervention.[76–78] NST of the IAN may be associated with a high incidence of false-positives and false-negatives (23% and 40%).[79,80] The first phase of NST involves first performing mechanoreceptive fiber testing (2-point discrimination, static light touch, directional discrimination). An uninvolved normal site should first be used as a baseline measurement. Marking can be done directly on the patient's face with erasable markers or by using photographs obtained before testing. When marking is done on the face, this must be photographed and kept for future reference and comparison.

Clinical NST begins with outlining the area of sensory disturbance (**Fig. 8**) using brush directional discrimination to differentiate normal and affected areas. Ideally, this is performed with a camel hair brush or a fine sable brush and the area is stroked at a constant rate. The patient is asked to give the direction of movement. The number of correct responses out of 10 is recorded. Static 2-point discrimination is performed next using any device that can reliably measure between 2 points. If the findings of brush stroke and 2-point discrimination are normal (level A testing), no further testing is required. The patient's injury is then diagnosed as a Sunderland first-degree injury. If findings are abnormal, level B testing should be performed. Level B testing (see **Fig. 8**) involves contact detection performed with either von-Frey hairs or Semmes-Weinstein monofilaments of multiple diameters that reflect the stiffness of the filament and the force required to deflect the fiber on contact. The narrowest fiber to be consistently detected by the patient and that requires the least force to detect is recorded from the control and affected sites. Level A and B testing assess the integrity of the large myelinated A-alpha and A-beta fiber types. If level B testing is normal, no further testing is required and the patient is considered a Sunderland second-degree injury. If findings are abnormal at level B, then testing proceeds to level C testing (pinprick nociception and thermal discrimination). Level C testing evaluates A-delta fibers and unmyelinated C fibers. A 30-gauze needle can be used to test for pin prick. Care should be taken not to injure the skin or oral mucosa. A yes or no is recorded as a response. Thermal detection can be performed with specialized Minnesota thermal discs or with hot or ice water on a cotton swab for suprathreshold thermal testing. This method has been shown to be valuable in iatrogenic injuries to the IAN and lingual nerve.[81] Normal responses at level C testing imply a moderate neurosensory impairment (Sunderland third-degree injury), whereas abnormal findings may either be consistent with severe nerve impairment with an increased thermal threshold versus a decreased nociceptive response (Sunderland fourth-degree injury) or lack of a response to pin prick or temperature (Sunderland fifth-degree injury).

Pain is a specific symptom to address during NST and can be recorded using a visual analog scale or with a more complex device such as the McGill pain questionnaire. Taste alteration to the distribution of the lingual nerve should also be assessed.[82]

MICRONEUROSURGERY FOR TRIGEMINAL NERVE INJURIES

Microneurosurgical procedures are best performed in the operating room under microscope

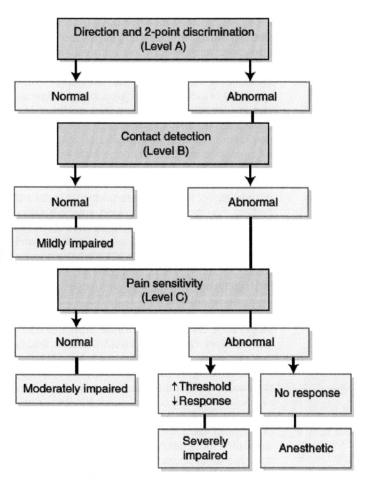

Fig. 8. Clinical NST algorithm. Level A testing (brush stroke direction and 2-point discrimination) is done first and, if normal, the examination is normal (Sunderland first-degree injury). If level A testing is abnormal, level B testing with contact detection is performed and, if normal, the examination indicates mild impairment (Sunderland second degree injury). If abnormal, level C testing (pinprick and thermal discrimination) is done and, if normal, the examination indicates moderate impairment (Sunderland third degree). If level C is abnormal, then the patient is either severely impaired (Sunderland fourth degree), or, with no response to testing, is considered anesthetic (Sunderland fifth degree). (*From* Schlieve T, Miloro M, and Kolokythas A. Chapter 5: Diagnosis and Management of Trigeminal and Facial Nerve Injuries. In: Fonseca, R, ed. Oral and Maxillofacial Surgery. 3rd ed. 2018: 70-113; with permission.)

or loupe magnification. In the setting of trauma, and with the absence of an existing laceration, surgical exposure for access to the IAN, lingual nerve, mandibular nerve, and ION is almost always preferred via an intraoral approach. This approach is preferred for ease of access but also offers the best esthetic result. The type of maxillofacial injury, surgeon experience, mechanism of injury, and location of injury should be considered when deciding on a surgical approach. In the setting of trauma, specific surgical approaches should be dictated by first preferred use of existing lacerations or an intraoral approach. In the setting of penetrating trauma or absence of an existing laceration, the lingual nerve may be approached using a paralingual or lingual gingival sulcus incision (**Fig. 9**). Distal IAN repairs may be accessed via a vestibular incision and lateral decortication of the IAN and MD (**Fig. 10**). The lateral wall should be decorticated 1 to 1.5 cm beyond the site of injury to mobilize the nerve for a tension-free repair. Alternatively, a transcervical approach may be used to access the IAN, which may be

useful for cases of limited mandibular opening. Alternatively, for proximal IAN injuries within the mandible, a sagittal split osteotomy may be performed as an alternative to lateral decortication to provide access (see **Fig. 10**). This approach provides excellent access to nerve injuries at or proximal to the second molar region of the mandible. In the absence of an existing laceration, access to the ION can usually be accomplished via a maxillary vestibule approach. Alternatively, and with more difficulty, access can also be accomplished by a lower lid incision or, in elderly patients with prominent wrinkles, an infraorbital incision. An osteotomy around the infraorbital canal may be needed to mobilize the nerve for repair.

After exposure, the nerve should carefully be dissected from the surrounding tissue bed. In the setting of trauma, this procedure, termed an external neurolysis, may be associated with significant scarring. This procedure may include microdissection of the nerve from surrounding tissues, or decortication from surround bone. External neurolysis in itself may be responsible for resolution of

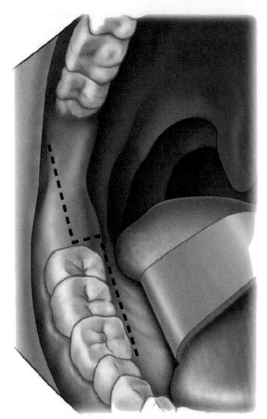

Fig. 9. Surgical access for lingual nerve repair using a lingual gingival sulcus approach (*dashed line*) with posterolateral extension. (*From* Miloro M, Kolokytas A. Chapter 25: Traumatic Injuries of the Trigeminal Nerve. In: Fonseca, R, ed. Oral and Maxillofacial Trauma. 4th ed. Elsevier; 2013: 650-682; with permission.)

neurosensory symptoms. Once external neurolysis is complete, the nerve and surrounding tissue should be examined for foreign material, bone or tooth fragments, or impinging surrounding anatomic structures. The site should carefully be debrided and thoroughly irrigated.

Internal neurolysis, or opening of the epineurium for fascicular examination, is indicated in cases where nerve continuity is maintained. There are several types of internal neurolysis described, including epifascicular epineurotomy, epifascicular epineurectomy, and intrafascicular epineurectomy. These types are of questionable benefit for the trigeminal nerve system and have to be weighed against the risk of further fibrosis and iatrogenic scarring.[83]

When neuroma is present, this should be excised, followed by restoration of nerve continuity. Neuroma should be excised from the proximal and distal nerve stumps until healthy nerve tissue is present. This procedure can be done in 1-mm increments until healthy nerve tissue is encountered (**Fig. 11**). Next, after mobilizing the nerve, if amendable, direct neurorrhaphy, epineural suturing with 3 to 4 8-0 or 9-0 nonabsorbable sutures (nylon) should be performed (**Fig. 12**). Coaptation is the alignment of individual fascicles during direct repair and is usually not possible with a polyfascicular nerve such as the trigeminal nerve. In the case of continuity defects, interpositional grafting is required in order to obtain a tension-free repair. This procedure is also required when mobilization of the nerve is not possible or will further compromise vitality of the nerve. Interpositional positional grafting may be performed using autograft donor sites such as the sural nerve or great auricular nerve and should be chosen based on diameter and fascicular pattern, and donor site morbidity and access. The sural nerve is the preferred graft site of the trigeminal system given that it closely matches the diameter and fascicular pattern of the trigeminal nerve system. The great auricular nerve is approximately 50% of the diameter of the trigeminal nerve and therefore may not be as useful and is limited to cable grafting (multiple grafts).

As an alternative to autograft, several other options exist, including alloplastic materials such as silastic, expanded polytetrafluoroethylene, polyester, polyglycolic acid polymer, autologous vein grafts, and allogenic nerve grafts, that can be used for entubulation techniques. Allogenic options are ideal because they eliminate the donor site morbidity. The use of allogenic nerve grafts in the repair of trigeminal nerve injuries resulting from iatrogenic injury and injury from pathologic resection has been well reported.[84] Given the rarity of this type of nerve injury,[85] its use in the traumatic setting has not been delineated.

THE FACIAL NERVE
Macroanatomy

The facial nerve has 3 distinct segments: (1) the intracranial, (2) intratemporal, and (3) extratemporal segments.

Intracranial Segment

The intracranial segment of the facial nerve is approximately 24 mm in length.[86,87]

The intracranial segment travels from the brainstem to the internal auditory canal (IAC) and contains 2 main components, the motor root and the nervus intermedius, which carries, sensory, preganglionic parasympathetic fibers and special afferent sensory fibers. These 2 components join just before becoming the intratemporal component of the facial nerve. The nervus intermedius provides sensation to the posterior concha and

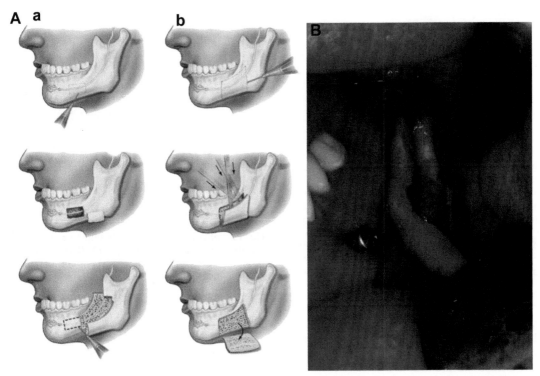

Fig. 10. (*A*) (a) Techniques for IAN access, including isolated decortication or a sagittal split osteotomy, with extension to the mental foramen if necessary. (b) Technique for wide access to the IAN via a complete lateral decortication window that may be replaced to protect the nerve repair site. ([*A*] *From* Miloro M, Kolokytas A. Chapter 25: Traumatic Injuries of the Trigeminal Nerve. In: Fonseca, R, ed. Oral and Maxillofacial Trauma. 4th ed. Elsevier; 2013: 650-682; with permission).

external auditory canal (EAC), taste sensation to the anterior two-thirds of the tongue, and secretomotor innervation of the minor salivary, submandibular, sublingual, and lacrimal glands.

Intratemporal Segment

The intratemporal segment of the facial nerve begins at the porus acusticus of the IAC and is divided into 4 portions as it travels to exit the stylomastoid foramen and becomes the extratemporal portion, including the first segment, the meatal portion (8–10 mm).[86,87] The second segment, the labyrinthine segment (3–5 mm) travels from the fundus to the geniculate ganglion. It is at this segment that the facial nerve runs through the narrowest portion of the IAC (0.68 mm) (**Fig. 13**).The labyrinthine ends at the geniculate ganglion and this is where the facial nerve gives off its first branch, the greater superficial petrosal nerve (**Fig. 14**), which carries preganglionic parasympathetic fibers from the superior salivatory nucleus to eventually innervate the lacrimal gland and minor salivary glands of the nose and palate.[88] The third segment is the tympanic segment, which extends from the geniculate ganglion to the second

genu and measures 8 to 11 mm (**Fig. 15**). This segment has the highest rate of bony dehiscence.[88,89] The fourth segment is the mastoid segment, and the nerve exits the temporal bone at the stylomastoid foramen 10 to 14 mm from the second genu (**Fig. 16**). It divides into the chorda tympani and innervates the stapedius muscle. After passing through the petrotympanic fissure and infratemporal fossa, the chorda tympani joins the lingual nerve before reaching the submandibular ganglion. Postganglionic fibers innervate the submandibular and sublingual glands, as well as providing taste sensation to the anterior two-thirds of the tongue.

Extratemporal Segment

This portion of the facial nerve begins at the stylomastoid foramen. The facial nerve gives off the posterior auricular nerve, which divides into the auricular and occipital branches innervating the auricularis posterior and occipital belly of the occipitofrontalis muscles respectively. After traveling between the digastric and stylohyoid muscles superficial to the styloid process, the facial nerve enters the substance of the parotid gland,

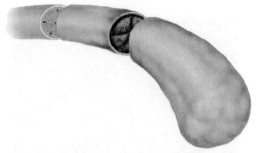

Fig. 11. Preparation of the nerve stump with serial 1.0-mm resections to remove scar tissue (neuroma) and ensure that normal-health neural tissue is encountered before the neurorrhaphy procedure. Failure to debride the nerve stumps adequately results in failure of neurosensory recover. (*From* Miloro M, Kolokytas A. Chapter 25: Traumatic Injuries of the Trigeminal Nerve. In: Fonseca, R, ed. Oral and Maxillofacial Trauma. 4th ed. Elsevier; 2013: 650-682; with permission.)

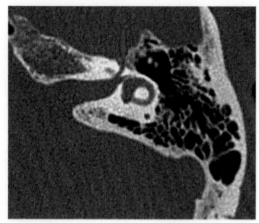

Fig. 13. Labyrinthine segment (fallopian canal) of the intratemporal facial nerve segment. Narrowest point (*arrow*) in the course of the facial nerve canal. (*From* Schlieve T, Miloro M, and Kolokythas A. Chapter 5: Diagnosis and Management of Trigeminal and Facial Nerve Injuries. In: Fonseca, R, ed. Oral and Maxillofacial Surgery. 3rd ed. 2018: 70-113; with permission.)

dividing the gland into the superficial and deep lobes. At an anatomic point located approximately 1.3 cm from the stylomastoid foramen, the facial nerve divides into its 2 main branches, the temporofacial and cervicofacial divisions. This point of division is termed the pes anserinus (Latin for goose foot).

The temporofacial and cervicofacial trunks then divide into the terminal 5 branches of the facial nerve (temporal, zygomatic, buccal, marginal mandibular, cervical) in varying patterns (**Fig. 17**). The temporal branch (possibly 2 branches) crosses the zygomatic arch within or deep to the temporoparietal fascia 0.8 to 3.5 cm anterior to the EAC[90,91] to innervate the frontalis, orbicularis

oculi, corrugator supercilii, and the anterior and superior auricular muscles, and serves as the efferent limb of the corneal reflex.

The zygomatic branch of the facial nerve exits the substance of the parotid gland approximately 3 cm anterior to the tragus and is located a mean vertical distance of 19 mm from a line connecting the lateral palpebral commissure and the tragus. It continues deep to the zygomaticus major and orbicularis oculi muscle to innervate the medial head of the orbital portion of the orbicularis oculi, depressor supercilii, and oblique head of the corrugator supercilii muscles.[92]

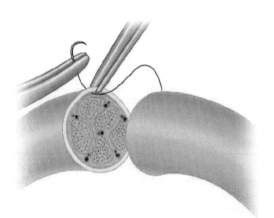

Fig. 12. Direct neurorrhaphy with epineurial sutures. (*From* Miloro M, Kolokytas A. Chapter 25: Traumatic Injuries of the Trigeminal Nerve. In: Fonseca, R, ed. Oral and Maxillofacial Trauma. 4th ed. Elsevier; 2013: 650-682; with permission.)

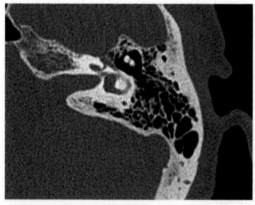

Fig. 14. Geniculate ganglion (*arrow*). (*From* Schlieve T, Miloro M, and Kolokythas A. Chapter 5: Diagnosis and Management of Trigeminal and Facial Nerve Injuries. In: Fonseca, R, ed. Oral and Maxillofacial Surgery. 3rd ed. 2018: 70-113; with permission.)

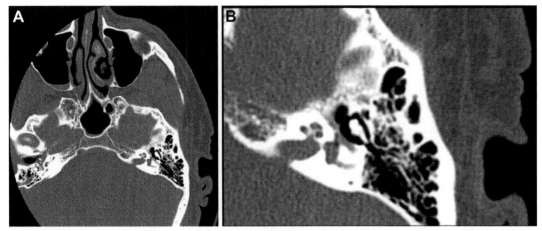

Fig. 15. (*A*) Tympanic segment of the intratemporal facial nerve (*green arrow*). (*B*) Magnified view of tympanic segment (*green line*). (*Courtesy of* Rui Fernandes, DMD, MD, Jacksonville, FL.)

The buccal branch of the facial nerve exits the anterior border parotid gland approximately 3 to 5 cm anterior to the tragus and along a line transverse to the axis of the zygomatic arch. The course of the buccal branch is always inferior to a line drawn from the tragus to the ala nasi.[93,94] The buccal branch provides innervation to the buccinator, levator labii superioris, risorius, levator labii superioris alaeque nasi, levator anguli oris, nasalis, orbicularis oris, depressor septi nasi, and procerus muscles.

The marginal mandibular branch of the facial nerve is the branch most commonly injured on surgical approaches to maxillofacial fractures. It innervates the depressor labii inferioris, depressor anguli oris, and mentalis muscles. The anatomy of the marginal branch has been extensively studied and, when anterior to the facial artery, the nerve is above the inferior border of the mandible in 100% of cases; however, when posterior to the facial artery, the nerve is above the inferior border of the mandible in 81% of cases. The nerve is superficial to the facial artery in 100% of cases.[95–97]

The cervical branch of the facial nerve innervates the platysma muscle. It is reliably located 1 cm below a line connecting the mastoid to the mentum at the position of the angle of the mandible.[98]

Microanatomy

The microanatomy of the facial nerve is very similar to that of the trigeminal nerve. It is a polyfascicular nerve, although it does not begin to show true fascicular organization until the geniculate ganglion. The number of fascicles varies depending on the motor branch.[99] The chorda

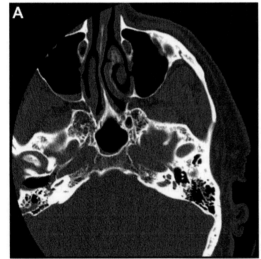

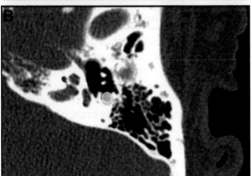

Fig. 16. (*A*) Mastoid segment of the intratemporal facial nerve segment (*red arrow*). (*B*) Magnified view of mastoid segment (*yellow circle*). (*Courtesy of* Rui Fernandes, DMD, MD, Jacksonville, FL.)

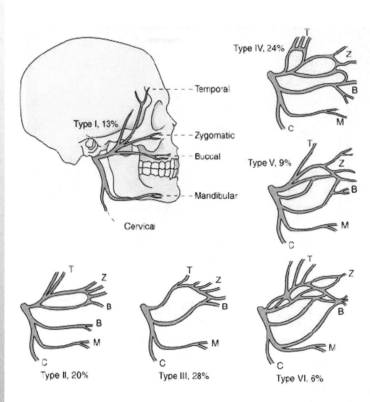

Fig. 17. Variations in the branching pattern of the facial nerve. (*From* Townsend C, Beauchamp RD, Evers BM, et al: Sabiston Textbook of Surgery, ed 19, St Louis, 2013, Saunders; with permission.)

tympani most commonly shows a monofascicular pattern before its fusion with the lingual nerve, where its fibers can no longer be recognized as separate entities.

Facial Nerve Imaging

MRI is the most common imaging entity used to assess injury to the facial nerve and is the preferred method of imaging to assess intracranial injury. For suspected injury to the intratemporal segment, which is common in the setting of facial trauma, a dedicated CT scan with thin cuts through the temporal bone is advocated. If disorder is suspected, the addition of MRI is advocated. When injury of the extracranial segment of the facial nerve is suspected, MRI is advocated.[88]

CT is the preferred imaging modality for injury or disorder of the intratemporal segment of the facial nerve. This modality should be dedicated high-resolution CT with thin cuts (0.6 mm) and helical acquisition. If disorder is suspected in addition to the trauma, contrast should be used. Alternatively in this scenario, MRI should be added. CT detects abnormal bony anatomy along the skull base that may indicate injury to the facial nerve, including disruption of the ossicles.

MRI is the preferred imaging modality for suspected neoplastic disorder of the intratemporal segment of the facial nerve and for injury to the intracranial and extratemporal segments of the facial nerve. The labyrinthine, cisternal, intracanalicular, and parotid segments of the facial nerve do not normally enhance on MRI, whereas the normal facial nerve faintly enhances in the geniculate ganglion, tympanic, and mastoid segments on gadolinium contrast MRI. Increased or asymmetric enhancement of these regions may indicate neoplastic or inflammatory processes. Once exiting the stylomastoid foramen, T1W axial views should be used to visualize the facial nerve. Ultrasonography is rarely used as routine imaging of the facial nerve.

Classification of Facial Nerve Injury

The House-Brackmann facial nerve functioning scale is the official grading scale of the Facial Nerve Disorders Committee of the Academy of Otolaryngology–Head and Neck Surgery (**Table 6**).[100] The House-Brackmann scale is of limited use in isolated injury to a single branch of the facial nerve. Many variation of the House-Brackmann scale have been described.[101]

MECHANISM OF INJURY TO THE FACIAL NERVE

Common causes of trigeminal nerve injury include Bell palsy (from a variety of causes), infection

Table 6	
The House-Brackmann facial nerve functioning scale	
Grade	**Description**
I	Normal facial function
II	Mild dysfunction. Slight weakness, slight synkinesis on close inspection. Moderate to good forehead function. Complete eye closure with minimal effort. Slight smile asymmetry with maximum effort. Normal symmetry and tone at rest
III	Moderate dysfunction. Obvious but not disfiguring difference between sides. Noticeable but not severe synkinesis. Slight to moderate forehead movement. Complete eye closure with effort. Strong but asymmetric smile with maximum effort. Normal symmetry and tone at rest
IV	Moderately severe dysfunction. Obvious weakness and/or disfiguring asymmetry. Severe synkinesis. No forehead movement. Incomplete eye closure. Asymmetric smile with maximum effort. Normal symmetry and tone at rest
V	Severe dysfunction. Barely perceptible motion. Synkinesis usually absent. No forehead movement. Incomplete eye closure. Slight movement at the corner of mouth. Asymmetry at rest
VI	Total paralysis. No movement

Adapted from House JW, Brackmann DE. Facial nerve grading system. Otolaryngol Head Neck Surg. 1985 Apr;93(2):146-7; with permission.

(most common is viral), and iatrogenic. Facial nerve injury in relation to trauma is discussed next.

Maxillofacial Trauma

The facial nerve can be injured by blunt or penetrating trauma, resulting in significant edema and compression, vascular compromise and ischemia, or transection. In addition, like the trigeminal nerve, the facial nerve can also be injured on surgical approaches to manage maxillofacial trauma. Facial trauma accounts for 15% of all cases of paralysis, with the most common cause being temporal bone fracture.

Temporal bone fractures can be divided into longitudinal and transverse in orientation. Often there are a mixture of the two. The longitudinal fracture of the temporal bone is the most common (70%–80%) and is characterized by a fracture line along the long axis of the petrous temporal bone. This line is the path of least resistance at the temporal bone. It is often associated with blunt trauma to the temporoparietal region. Only 10% to 20% of longitudinal fractures are associated with facial nerve injury, with 94% remaining as permanent.[102,103] Transverse fractures extend perpendicular to the long axis of the petrous, often from the jugular foramen or foramen magnum to the middle cranial fossa and involve the bony labyrinth and/or geniculate ganglion. In the case of bony labyrinth involvement, sensorial hearing loss and vertigo are common. These fractures result from high impact to the frontal or occipital bone, and up to 50% have facial nerve injury, which is often permanent.[102,103] Prognosis is improved for patients with delayed paralysis because this is often associated with edema. Treatment of facial nerve injury associated with temporal bone fracture should be guided by the facial nerve conduction examination. If indicated, facial nerve decompression should be performed as soon as possible (within 1 month from injury).[104] Extratemporal facial nerve injury should be evaluated and managed to avoid long-term functional and cosmetic deficits. In general, injuries proximal to a vertical line descending from the lateral canthus are amendable to surgical repair.[105]

Clinical Evaluation of Facial Nerve Injuries

The physical examination should include a thorough head and neck examination, noting any facial asymmetry or lacerations. Symptoms such as pain, dizziness, changes in hearing, hyperacusis, tinnitus, and changes in taste should be noted. Otoscopy should be completed to check for EAC lacerations, step-offs, hemotympanum, otorrhea, or tympanic membrane perforation. When cerebrospinal fluid leak is suspected, fluid should be collected and sent for beta-2 transferrin testing. Facial nerve conduction testing with topographic and electrodiagnostic methods may be helpful to determine the site and severity of injury as well as to help decide the proposed treatment and ideal management.[106] Facial nerve testing is divided into 2 categories: topographic testing (Schirmer test, stapedius reflex testing, and taste test) and electrodiagnostic testing, which includes nerve excitability testing, maximal stimulation testing, electroneurography, and electromyography. All electrodiagnostic tests require a normal contralateral facial nerve for comparison.

Treatment of Traumatic Extratemporal Facial Nerve Injuries

Penetrating injuries account for most extratemporal nerve injuries seen in the traumatic setting. Prompt and expeditious recognition and management afford the best long-term prognosis. Repair within 72 hours of injury allows nerve stimulation to identify cut distal nerve endings. Beyond 72 hours, motor end-plate depolarization is not possible because neurotransmitter stores are depleted. Repair within 30 days offers the greatest probability of success.[107] Loupe or operating microscope magnification is advised for identifying neural structures. Access via preexisting incisions or lacerations is always preferred. In the case of delayed repair, a transfacial approach such as that used for parotid surgery (modified Blair) is preferred. As with the standard approach with superficial parotidectomy, the main trunk of the facial nerve should be identified using standard landmarks. The course of the facial nerve should be dissected distal until the site of injury is identified (**Fig. 18**). Performing a superficial parotidectomy may assist the surgeon in performing a tension-free repair (**Fig. 19**). Once identified, the proximal and distal ends should be dissected free to about 5 to 10 mm. Electrical stimulation can be applied. In the presence of a good response, further exploration is not required. In the absence of a good

response, formal repair should take place. In the case of proximal injuries, decompression of the nerve from the mastoid and temporal bones can provide additional mobilization of the facial nerve.[108]

When tension-free repair is not possible, interposition (cable) grafts should be considered, which can be in the form of autograft, such as great auricular, sural, medial antebrachial, or lateral antebrachial cutaneous nerves. Unlike in trigeminal nerve autografting, the great auricular nerve is preferred because of its similar size to the facial nerve branches and proximity to the recipient site. If a graft of more than 8 to 10 cm is needed, an alternative donor site, such as the sural nerve, should be used. If the facial nerve stump is unavailable, a cross-facial graft can be considered using the contralateral facial nerve and nerve graft.[109] Cross-face nerve grafting carries the benefit of borrowing nerves with similar functions and can allow spontaneous and emotional facial expression without dyskinesis. If the contralateral facial nerve is not available, a

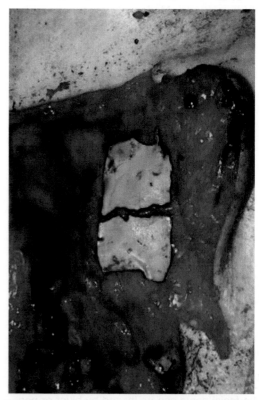

Fig. 19. Repaired facial nerve branch. (*From* Schlieve T, Miloro M, and Kolokythas A. Chapter 5: Diagnosis and Management of Trigeminal and Facial Nerve Injuries. In: Fonseca, R, ed. Oral and Maxillofacial Surgery. 3rd ed. 2018: 70-113; with permission.)

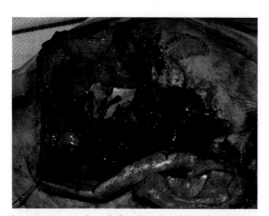

Fig. 18. Proximal and distal ends of the facial nerve identified and isolated. (*From* Schlieve T, Miloro M, and Kolokythas A. Chapter 5: Diagnosis and Management of Trigeminal and Facial Nerve Injuries. In: Fonseca, R, ed. Oral and Maxillofacial Surgery. 3rd ed. 2018: 70-113; with permission.)

nerve crossover or nerve transfer may be performed. Common donor nerves include the ipsilateral masseter branch of the trigeminal nerve and partial hypoglossal nerve.[110,111]

A Note on Dysesthesias

For management of persistent pain and neurosensory disturbance to the IAN, data can be extracted from the dental implant literature.[112] Management should be symptom driven. Patients with neurosensory disturbances (eg, neuropathic pain, complex regional pain syndrome) and dysesthesia should be managed differently than those with neurosensory disturbance alone. Traumatic dysesthesia of the trigeminal nerve may be treated with capsaicin, a substance P depletion medication.[113] Initial therapy should focus on pharmacologic management rather than invasive procedures. In addition, psychological and behavioral management should be considered. Consultation to psychology, social work, neurology, and pain specialists should be considered in refractory dysesthesias.

Initially in the setting of dysesthesia, treatment should be focused on suppressing the inflammatory process. Treatment of neuropathic pain should be focused on reducing levels of cytokines, chemokines, and inflammatory mediators, such as interleukin-1b and tumor necrosis factor.[114] Therefore, initial management should include antiinflammatory drugs such as steroids and nonsteroidal antiinflammatory drugs. In the acute phase, corticosteroids should be considered because they may prevent the development of neuroma.[115] In the presence of nerve compression, 1 to 2 mL of dexamethasone (4 mg/mL) should be applied topically to minimize neural inflammation and soft tissue swelling that could compress the nerve. In addition, an oral regimen of dexamethasone should be administered for 6 days.[115]

Antidepressants and anticonvulsants are available alternatives in the management of neuropathic pain.[116] Tricyclic antidepressants drugs, such as amitriptyline, desipramine, and nortriptyline, work on neuropathic pain via an analgesic effect, rather than their antidepressant effect. Tricyclic antidepressants inhibit the reuptake of monoamines with a blockade of sodium channels. In addition, tricyclic antidepressants have anticholinergic effects. Serotonin and norepinephrine reuptake inhibitors, such as venlafaxine and duloxetine, may also be used to managed neuropathic pain. Gabapentin and pregabalin, two commonly used anticonvulsant drugs, may be used in the management of neuropathic pain. They work by decreasing nociceptive transmission and central sensitization. Patients must be forewarned of the sedative effects of gabapentin.

SUMMARY

The trigeminal and facial nerve systems, and the structures that they innervate, are almost always involved in the setting of craniomaxillofacial trauma. Nerve injuries must be first identified, assessed, and classified by a thorough and systematic physical examination. Imaging should be prudent, expeditious, and used as an adjunct to the clinical examination. If indicated, repair of nerve injuries should be performed as soon as possible for improved outcomes. Systematic and regular preoperative and postoperative clinical examinations provide the best estimate of clinical recovery following nerve injury.

CLINICS CARE POINTS

- Surgeons should attempt to retrieve preinjury imaging and compare with imaging taken after nerve injury. This comparison includes, but is not limited to, CT, MRI, and panoramic radiographs.
- Clinical NST should be done in a quiet, controlled environment and performed in a similar standardized way at each evaluation.
- MRI, or, if available, MRN is the preferred image modality when assessing the nerve itself. CT is preferred for assessing the hard tissues surrounding the nerve.
- Dysesthesias are often best managed with nonsurgical treatment, and consultation with other specialties such as pain specialists and neurologists may be helpful.

DISCLOSURE

Drs M. Miloro and M.R. Markiewicz are consultants for AxoGen (Alachua, FL).

REFERENCES

1. Anderson LC, Kosinski TF, Mentag PJ. A review of the intraosseous course of the nerves of the mandible. J Oral Implantol 1991;17:394–403.
2. Gowgiel JM. The position and course of the mandibular canal. J Oral Implantol 1992;18:383–5.
3. Stella JP, Tharanon W. A precise radiographic method to determine the location of the inferior alveolar canal in the posterior edentulous

mandible: implications for dental implants. Part 2: Clinical application. Int J Oral Maxillofac Implants 1990;5:23–9.

4. Cutright B, Quillopa N, Schubert W. An anthropometric analysis of the key foramina for maxillofacial surgery. J Oral Maxillofac Surg 2003;61:354–7.

5. Hu KS, Yun HS, Hur MS, et al. Branching patterns and intraosseous course of the mental nerve. J Oral Maxillofac Surg 2007;65:2288–94.

6. Kim SY, Hu KS, Chung IH, et al. Topographic anatomy of the lingual nerve and variations in communication pattern of the mandibular nerve branches. Surg Radiol Anat 2004;26:128–35.

7. Miloro M, Halkias LE, Slone HW, et al. Assessment of the lingual nerve in the third molar region using magnetic resonance imaging. J Oral Maxillofac Surg 1997;55:134–7.

8. Kiesselbach JE, Chamberlain JG. Clinical and anatomic observations on the relationship of the lingual nerve to the mandibular third molar region. J Oral Maxillofac Surg 1984;42:565–7.

9. Erdogmus S, Govsa F, Celik S. Anatomic position of the lingual nerve in the mandibular third molar region as potential risk factors for nerve palsy. J Craniofac Surg 2008;19:264–70.

10. Pogrel MA, Le H. Etiology of lingual nerve injuries in the third molar region: a cadaver and histologic study. J Oral Maxillofac Surg 2006;64:1790–4.

11. Karakas P, Uzel M, Koebke J. The relationship of the lingual nerve to the third molar region using radiographic imaging. Br Dent J 2007;203:29–31.

12. Holzle FW, Wolff KD. Anatomic position of the lingual nerve in the mandibular third molar region with special consideration of an atrophied mandibular crest: an anatomical study. Int J Oral Maxillofac Surg 2001;30:333–8.

13. Behnia H, Kheradvar A, Shahrokhi M. An anatomic study of the lingual nerve in the third molar region. J Oral Maxillofac Surg 2000;58:649–51. discussion 652-643.

14. Pogrel MA, Renaut A, Schmidt B, et al. The relationship of the lingual nerve to the mandibular third molar region: an anatomic study. J Oral Maxillofac Surg 1995;53:1178–81.

15. Skandalakis JE, Gray SW, Rowe JS Jr. Surgical anatomy of the submandibular triangle. Am Surg 1979;45:590–6.

16. Zahm DS, Munger BL. The innervation of the primate fungiform papilla–development, distribution and changes following selective ablation. Brain Res 1985;356:147–86.

17. Aziz SR, Marchena JM, Puran A. Anatomic characteristics of the infraorbital foramen: a cadaver study. J Oral Maxillofac Surg 2000;58:992–6.

18. Hu KS, Kwak J, Koh KS, et al. Topographic distribution area of the infraorbital nerve. Surg Radiol Anat 2007;29:383–8.

19. Friede RL, Bischhausen R. The organization of endoneural collagen in peripheral nerves as revealed with the scanning electron microscope. J Neurol Sci 1978;38:83–8.

20. Ushiki T, Ide C. Three-dimensional architecture of the endoneurium with special reference to the collagen fibril arrangement in relation to nerve fibers. Arch Histol Jpn 1986;49:553–63.

21. Mozsary PG, Middleton RA. Microsurgical reconstruction of the infraorbital nerves. J Oral Maxillofac Surg 1983;41:697–700.

22. Svane TJ, Wolford LM, Milam SB, et al. Fascicular characteristics of the human inferior alveolar nerve. J Oral Maxillofac Surg 1986;44:431–4.

23. Girod SC, Neukam FW, Girod B, et al. The fascicular structure of the lingual nerve and the chorda tympani: an anatomic study. J Oral Maxillofac Surg 1989;47:607–9.

24. Smoliar E, Smoliar A, Sorkin L, et al. Microcirculatory bed of the human trigeminal nerve. Anat Rec 1998;250:245–9.

25. Lundborg G. Intraneural microcirculation. Orthop Clin North Am 1988;19:1–12.

26. Miloro M, Kolokythas A. Inferior alveolar and lingual nerve imaging. Atlas Oral Maxillofac Surg Clin North Am 2011;19:35–46.

27. Qian J, Herrera JJ, Narayana PA. Neuronal and axonal degeneration in experimental spinal cord injury: in vivo proton magnetic resonance spectroscopy and histology. J Neurotrauma 2010;27:599–610.

28. Aagaard BD, Maravilla KR, Kliot M. MR neurography. MR imaging of peripheral nerves. Magn Reson Imaging Clin N Am 1998;6:179–94.

29. Cudlip SA, Howe FA, Griffiths JR, et al. Magnetic resonance neurography of peripheral nerve following experimental crush injury, and correlation with functional deficit. J Neurosurg 2002;96:755–9.

30. Grant GA, Goodkin R, Maravilla KR, et al. MR neurography: diagnostic utility in the surgical treatment of peripheral nerve disorders. Neuroimaging Clin N Am 2004;14:115–33.

31. Hatipoglu HG, Durakoglugil T, Ciliz D, et al. Comparison of FSE T2W and 3D FIESTA sequences in the evaluation of posterior fossa cranial nerves with MR cisternography. Diagn Interv Radiol 2007;13:56–60.

32. Filler AG, Kliot M, Howe FA, et al. Application of magnetic resonance neurography in the evaluation of patients with peripheral nerve pathology. J Neurosurg 1996;85:299–309.

33. Filler AG, Maravilla KR, Tsuruda JS. MR neurography and muscle MR imaging for image diagnosis of disorders affecting the peripheral nerves and musculature. Neurol Clin 2004;22:643–82. vi-vii.

34. Furuya Y, Ryu H, Uemura K, et al. MRI of intracranial neurovascular compression. J Comput Assist Tomogr 1992;16:503–5.

35. Rocca MA, Filippi M. Functional MRI in multiple sclerosis. J Neuroimaging 2007;17(Suppl 1): 36S–41S.

36. McDonald AR, Roberts TP, Rowley HA, et al. Noninvasive somatosensory monitoring of the injured inferior alveolar nerve using magnetic source imaging. J Oral Maxillofac Surg 1996;54:1068–72. discussion 1072-1064.

37. Burian E, Sollmann N, Ritschl LM, et al. High resolution MRI for quantitative assessment of inferior alveolar nerve impairment in course of mandible fractures: an imaging feasibility study. Sci Rep 2020;10:11566.

38. Parker GD, Harnsberger HR. Clinical-radiologic issues in perineural tumor spread of malignant diseases of the extracranial head and neck. Radiographics 1991;11:383–99.

39. Huisman M, Staruch RM, Ladouceur-Wodzak M, et al. Non-invasive targeted peripheral nerve ablation using 3D MR neurography and MRI-guided high-intensity focused ultrasound (MR-HIFU): pilot study in a swine model. PLoS One 2015;10: e0144742.

40. Aagaard BD, Maravilla KR, Kliot M. Magnetic resonance neurography: magnetic resonance imaging of peripheral nerves. Neuroimaging Clin N Am 2001;11(1):viii, 131-146.

41. Merlini L, Viallon M, De Coulon G, et al. MRI neurography and diffusion tensor imaging of a sciatic perineuroma in a child. Pediatr Radiol 2008;38: 1009–12.

42. Tsuchiya K, Imai M, Tateishi H, et al. Neurography of the spinal nerve roots by diffusion tensor scanning applying motion-probing gradients in six directions. Magn Reson Med Sci 2007;6:1–5.

43. Wessig C, Jestaedt L, Sereda MW, et al. Gadofluorine M-enhanced magnetic resonance nerve imaging: comparison between acute inflammatory and chronic degenerative demyelination in rats. Exp Neurol 2008;210:137–43.

44. Sunderland S. A classification of peripheral nerve injuries producing loss of function. Brain 1951;74: 491–516.

45. Sunderland S. Observations on the treatment of traumatic injuries of peripheral nerves. Br J Surg 1947;35:36–42.

46. Wyrick JD, Stern PJ. Secondary nerve reconstruction. Hand Clin 1992;8:587–98.

47. Mackinnon SE. Surgical management of the peripheral nerve gap. Clin Plast Surg 1989;16: 587–603.

48. Rosen B, Lundborg G. A model instrument for the documentation of outcome after nerve repair. J Hand Surg Am 2000;25:535–43.

49. Stoll G, Muller HW. Nerve injury, axonal degeneration and neural regeneration: basic insights. Brain Pathol 1999;9:313–25.

50. Muller HW, Stoll G. Nerve injury and regeneration: basic insights and therapeutic interventions. Curr Opin Neurol 1998;11:557–62.

51. Forman DS, Wood DK, DeSilva S. Rate of regeneration of sensory axons in transected rat sciatic nerve repaired with epineurial sutures. J Neurol Sci 1979;44:55–9.

52. Hanz S, Fainzilber M. Retrograde signaling in injured nerve–the axon reaction revisited. J Neurochem 2006;99:13–9.

53. Bisby MA. Changes in the composition of labeled protein transported in motor axons during their regeneration. J Neurobiol 1980;11:435–45.

54. McQuarrie IG. The effect of a conditioning lesion on the regeneration of motor axons. Brain Res 1978; 152:597–602.

55. Mc IA, Bradley K, Brock LG. Responses of motoneurons undergoing chromatolysis. J Gen Physiol 1959;42:931–58.

56. Brody H, Rodbard S. Chromatolysis and vacuolation of specific diencephalic nuclei induced by acute pyrexia. Am J Physiol 1959;196:33–5.

57. Lavelle A, Lavelle FW. Neuronal swelling and chromatolysis as influenced by the state of cell development. Am J Anat 1958;102:219–41.

58. Causey G, Stratmann CJ. Changes in the nucleic acid content of ganglion cells during chromatolysis and after stimulation. Biochem J 1956;64:29–32.

59. Campbell B. Chromatolysis and the model of the neurone. J Physiol 1954;124:28–29P.

60. Terry RD, Harkin JC. Wallerian degeneration and regeneration of peripheral nerves. Prog Neurobiol 1959;4:303–20.

61. Goodrum JF, Bouldin TW. The cell biology of myelin degeneration and regeneration in the peripheral nervous system. J Neuropathol Exp Neurol 1996; 55:943–53.

62. Nathaniel EJ, Pease DC. Regenerative changes in rat dorsal roots following Walerian degeneration. J Ultrastruct Res 1963;52:533–49.

63. Yang DP, Zhang DP, Mak KS, et al. Schwann cell proliferation during Wallerian degeneration is not necessary for regeneration and remyelination of the peripheral nerves: axon-dependent removal of newly generated Schwann cells by apoptosis. Mol Cell Neurosci 2008;38:80–8.

64. Bajestan SN, Umehara F, Shirahama Y, et al. Desert hedgehog-patched 2 expression in peripheral nerves during Wallerian degeneration and regeneration. J Neurobiol 2006;66:243–55.

65. Otsu A. Neurohistological researches of peripheral nerves of some pathological materials. (Degeneration and regeneration). Acta Neuroveg (Wien) 1962;22:312–32.

66. Munger BL, Renehan WE. Degeneration and regeneration of peripheral nerve in the rat trigeminal system: III. Abnormal sensory reinnervation of

rat guard hairs following nerve transection and crush. J Comp Neurol 1989;283:169–76.

67. Stoll G, Jander S, Myers RR. Degeneration and regeneration of the peripheral nervous system: from Augustus Waller's observations to neuroinflammation. J Peripher Nerv Syst 2002;7:13–27.

68. Wisniewski HM. Difference in the morphology of Wallerian degeneration in the central nervous system (CNS) and peripheral nervous system (PNS) and its effect on regeneration. Birth Defects Orig Artic Ser 1983;19:389–95.

69. Renzi G, Carboni A, Perugini M, et al. Posttraumatic trigeminal nerve impairment: a prospective analysis of recovery patterns in a series of 103 consecutive facial fractures. J Oral Maxillofac Surg 2004;62:1341–6.

70. Schultze-Mosgau S, Erbe M, Rudolph D, et al. Prospective study on post-traumatic and postoperative sensory disturbances of the inferior alveolar nerve and infraorbital nerve in mandibular and midfacial fractures. J Craniomaxillofac Surg 1999;27:86–93.

71. Lee SY, Kim SH, Hwang JH, et al. Sensory recovery after infraorbital nerve avulsion injury. Arch Craniofac Surg 2020;21:244–8.

72. Yu H, Shen G, Wang X, et al. Navigation-guided reduction and orbital floor reconstruction in the treatment of zygomatic-orbital-maxillary complex fractures. J Oral Maxillofac Surg 2010;68:28–34.

73. Marchena JM, Padwa BL, Kaban LB. Sensory abnormalities associated with mandibular fractures: incidence and natural history. J Oral Maxillofac Surg 1998;56:822–5. discussion 825-826.

74. Iizuka T, Lindqvist C. Sensory disturbances associated with rigid internal fixation of mandibular fractures. J Oral Maxillofac Surg 1991;49:1264–8.

75. Robinson PP. Observations on the recovery of sensation following inferior alveolar nerve injuries. Br J Oral Maxillofac Surg 1988;26:177–89.

76. Fogaca WC, Fereirra MC, Dellon AL. Infraorbital nerve injury associated with zygoma fractures: documentation with neurosensory testing. Plast Reconstr Surg 2004;113:834–8.

77. Ghali GE, Epker BN. Clinical neurosensory testing: practical applications. J Oral Maxillofac Surg 1989; 47:1074–8.

78. Kalladka M, Viswanath A, Gomes J, et al. Trigeminal nerve injury following accidental airbag deployment and assessment with quantitative sensory testing. Cranio 2007;25:138–43.

79. Zuniga JR, Meyer RA, Gregg JM, et al. The accuracy of clinical neurosensory testing for nerve injury diagnosis. J Oral Maxillofac Surg 1998;56:2–8.

80. Ziccardi VB, Hullett JS, Gomes J. Physical neurosensory testing versus current perception threshold assessment in trigeminal nerve injuries related to dental treatment: a retrospective study. Quintessence Int 2009;40:603–9.

81. Renton T, Thexton A, Hankins M, et al. Quantitative thermosensory testing of the lingual and inferior alveolar nerves in health and after iatrogenic injury. Br J Oral Maxillofac Surg 2003;41:36–42.

82. Hillerup S, Hjorting-Hansen E, Reumert T. Repair of the lingual nerve after iatrogenic injury: a follow-up study of return of sensation and taste. J Oral Maxillofac Surg 1994;52:1028–31.

83. Ziccardi VB, Steinberg MJ. Timing of trigeminal nerve microsurgery: a review of the literature. J Oral Maxillofac Surg 2007;65:1341–5.

84. Salomon D, Miloro M, Kolokythas A. Outcomes of immediate allograft reconstruction of long-span defects of the inferior alveolar nerve. J Oral Maxillofac Surg 2016;74:2507–14.

85. Zuniga JR. Sensory outcomes after reconstruction of lingual and inferior alveolar nerve discontinuities using processed nerve allograft–a case series. J Oral Maxillofac Surg 2015;73:734–44.

86. Feng Y, Zhang YQ, Liu M, et al. Sectional anatomy aid for improvement of decompression surgery approach to vertical segment of facial nerve. J Craniofac Surg 2012;23:906–8.

87. White H, Rosenthal E. Static and dynamic repairs of facial nerve injuries. Oral Maxillofac Surg Clin North Am 2013;25:303–12.

88. Gupta S, Mends F, Hagiwara M, et al. Imaging the facial nerve: a contemporary review. Radiol Res Pract 2013;2013:248039.

89. Nager GT, Proctor B. Anatomic variations and anomalies involving the facial canal. Otolaryngol Clin North Am 1991;24:531–53.

90. Al-Kayat A, Bramley P. A modified pre-auricular approach to the temporomandibular joint and malar arch. Br J Oral Surg 1979;17:91–103.

91. Miloro M, Redlinger S, Pennington DM, et al. In situ location of the temporal branch of the facial nerve. J Oral Maxillofac Surg 2007;65:2466–9.

92. Saylam C, Ucerler H, Orhan M, et al. Anatomic guides to precisely localize the zygomatic branches of the facial nerve. J Craniofac Surg 2006;17:50–3.

93. Pogrel MA, Schmidt B, Ammar A. The relationship of the buccal branch of the facial nerve to the parotid duct. J Oral Maxillofac Surg 1996;54:71–3.

94. Saylam C, Ucerler H, Orhan M, et al. Anatomic landmarks of the buccal branches of the facial nerve. Surg Radiol Anat 2006;28:462–7.

95. Dingman RO, Grabb WC. Surgical anatomy of the mandibular ramus of the facial nerve based on the dissection of 100 facial halves. Plast Reconstr Surg Transplant Bull 1962;29:266–72.

96. Rodel R, Lang J. [Peripheral branches of the facial nerve in the cheek and chin area. Anatomy and clinical consequences]. HNO 1996;44:572–6.

97. Batra AP, Mahajan A, Gupta K. Marginal mandibular branch of the facial nerve: An anatomical study. Indian J Plast Surg 2010;43:60–4.

98. Chowdhry S, Yoder EM, Cooperman RD, et al. Locating the cervical motor branch of the facial nerve: anatomy and clinical application. Plast Reconstr Surg 2010;126:875–9.

99. Captier G, Canovas F, Bonnel F, et al. Organization and microscopic anatomy of the adult human facial nerve: anatomical and histological basis for surgery. Plast Reconstr Surg 2005;115:1457–65.

100. House JW, Brackmann DE. Facial nerve grading system. Otolaryngol Head Neck Surg 1985;93: 146–7.

101. Alicandri-Ciufelli M, Pavesi G, Presutti L. Facial nerve grading scales: systematic review of the literature and suggestion for uniformity. Plast Reconstr Surg 2015;135:929e–30e.

102. Chang CY, Cass SP. Management of facial nerve injury due to temporal bone trauma. Am J Otol 1999;20:96–114.

103. Liu Y, Han J, Zhou X, et al. Surgical management of facial paralysis resulting from temporal bone fractures. Acta Otolaryngol 2014;134:656–60.

104. Kim J, Moon IS, Shim DB, et al. The effect of surgical timing on functional outcomes of traumatic facial nerve paralysis. J Trauma 2010;68:924–9.

105. Rovak JM, Tung TH, Mackinnon SE. The surgical management of facial nerve injury. Semin Plast Surg 2004;18:23–30.

106. Gantz BJ, Gmuer AA, Holliday M, et al. Electroneurographic evaluation of the facial nerve. Method and technical problems. Ann Otol Rhinol Laryngol 1984;93:394–8.

107. Bascom DA, Schaitkin BM, May M, et al. Facial nerve repair: a retrospective review. Facial Plast Surg 2000;16:309–13.

108. Piza-Katzer H, Balogh B, Muzika-Herczeg E, et al. Secondary end-to-end repair of extensive facial nerve defects: surgical technique and postoperative functional results. Head Neck 2004;26:770–7.

109. Morley SE. Combining an end to side nerve to masseter transfer with cross face nerve graft for functional upgrade in partial facial paralysis-an observational cohort study. J Plast Reconstr Aesthet Surg 2020.

110. Ueda K, Akiyoshi K, Suzuki Y, et al. Combination of hypoglossal-facial nerve jump graft by end-to-side neurorrhaphy and cross-face nerve graft for the treatment of facial paralysis. J Reconstr Microsurg 2007;23:181–7.

111. Gibelli D, Tarabbia F, Restelli S, et al. Three-dimensional assessment of restored smiling mobility after reanimation of unilateral facial palsy by triple innervation technique. Int J Oral Maxillofac Surg 2020; 49:536–42.

112. Al-Sabbagh M, Okeson JP, Bertoli E, et al. Persistent pain and neurosensory disturbance after dental implant surgery: prevention and treatment. Dent Clin North Am 2015;59:143–56.

113. Canavan D, Graff-Radford SB, Gratt BM. Traumatic dysesthesia of the trigeminal nerve. J Orofac Pain 1994;8:391–6.

114. Costigan M, Scholz J, Woolf CJ. Neuropathic pain: a maladaptive response of the nervous system to damage. Annu Rev Neurosci 2009;32:1–32.

115. Misch CE, Resnik R. Mandibular nerve neurosensory impairment after dental implant surgery: management and protocol. Implant Dent 2010;19: 378–86.

116. Park JH, Lee SH, Kim ST. Pharmacologic management of trigeminal nerve injury pain after dental implant surgery. Int J Prosthodont 2010;23:342–6.

Management of Scalp Injuries

Joshua Yoon, MD[a,b], Joseph S. Puthumana, BA[c], Arthur J. Nam, MD, MS[a,*]

KEYWORDS

- Scalp trauma • Scalp cancer • Scalp ablation • Scalp injury • Reconstruction

KEY POINTS

- Knowledge of the scalp soft tissue layers and neurovasculature are integral in understanding anatomic limitations/considerations and reconstruction planning.
- The goal of scalp reconstruction is to provide durable soft tissue coverage that restores normal contours and appearance of hair-bearing areas.
- The reconstruction modality is determined by wound location, size, depth, presence of calvarial defects, previous or planned radiation, chronic infections, prior surgeries, and need for oncologic surveillance.

INTRODUCTION

Scalp defects secondary to trauma and oncologic resections pose challenges to reconstructive surgeons not only due to the size, depth, location, and configuration of the wound but also because of hair pattern and presence of concomitant injuries (eg, cranial fractures, closed head injuries), prior surgeries, and/or previous radiation therapy.[1,2] In traumatic scalp wounds, the mechanism of injuries can vary from falls and assaults to burns and hair entrapment in industrial machines. Similarly, the extent of scalp injuries can vary from simple lacerations to complex avulsions or defects.[3–5] In addition to soft tissues, calvarial defects from oncologic resections may also be present, and these defects are usually readily visible and can be disfiguring, which can cause social and psychological stress, thereby negatively affecting quality of life.[6]

One of the first documented experiences in the management of scalp injuries was in the late 1600s by Augustin Belloste.[7] Since that time, the management and the means for reconstruction of scalp injuries have progressed significantly to address both appropriate soft tissue coverage and also optimizing aesthetic results. However, despite these advancements, methods for scalp reconstruction can still be imperfect and provide suboptimal results, which is largely driven by anatomic factors and difficulty replicating and/or replacing hair-bearing areas. Thus careful preoperative planning and discussions must be had with the patient to counsel on both complications such as soft tissue necrosis, scar complications, alopecia, and skin pigmentation and/or texture changes, in addition to the expectations for aesthetic outcomes.[1] The surgeon's surgical armamentarium should be well equipped with up-to-date management strategies and surgical techniques for different types of scalp defects. The purpose of this review is to discuss different surgical strategies to address various scalp defects.

[a] Division of Plastic, Reconstructive & Maxillofacial Surgery, R Adams Cowley Shock Trauma Center, University of Maryland School of Medicine, 110 South Paca Street, Room 4S-125, Baltimore, MD 21201, USA; [b] Department of Surgery, George Washington University Hospital, Washington, DC, USA; [c] R Adams Cowley Shock Trauma Center, University of Maryland School of Medicine, 110 South Paca Street, Room 4S-125, Baltimore, MD 21201, USA
* Corresponding author.
E-mail address: anam@som.umaryland.edu

Oral Maxillofacial Surg Clin N Am 33 (2021) 407–416
https://doi.org/10.1016/j.coms.2021.05.001

ANATOMY
Soft Tissues

The scalp consists of 5 distinct tissue layers and is commonly remembered by the mnemonic: SCALP (**S**kin, sub**C**utaneous layer, **A**poneurotic (galea) layer, **L**oose areolar tissue, **P**ericranium) (**Fig. 1**). The outermost layer is the skin (ie, epidermis and dermis), which is generally thicker than most other areas of skin. The thickness ranges from 3 to 8 mm and will depend on the density of hair: the densest areas have the thickest skin, and the less dense or alopecic areas have the thinnest. Hair follicles, sebaceous glands, and sweat glands are found in this layer. The second layer is the subcutaneous layer where the extensive complex network of blood vessels, lymphatics, and nerves reside. There are also fibrous septa that partition the fat into small compartments. The aponeurotic layer (eg, galea aponeurotica) is also referred to as the epicranial aponeurosis. The galea is a durable fibrous aponeurosis that is resistant to stretching and is densely adherent to the subcutaneous tissues. This fibrous layer spans between the insertions of the frontalis and occipitalis muscles, and laterally toward the temporal fascia, and is considered the "strength layer." The fourth layer is the loose areolar tissue layer, which is also known as the subgaleal compartment or innominate fascia. As the name implies, this layer is composed of filmy loose areolar tissue and is mostly avascular; however, emissary veins are contained within this layer. This layer is important because not only does it provide scalp mobility but it is amenable to surgical dissection without disrupting blood flow to the skin, thus allowing for large flaps to be safely raised. The last layer is the pericranium, which is similar to the galea in structure; however, it is very thin and located directly over the skull.[8,9]

Vascular Anatomy

The primary blood supply for the scalp is derived from both internal and external carotid arteries and travels within the subcutaneous layer (**Fig. 2**). The blood supply can be described as a centripetally distributed system where larger vessels are found in the periphery and then branch medially and centrally leading to an extensive collateralized vascular system. These arteries are found in the deep layers of the dermis and are adherent to the dermis. The scalp has been traditionally divided into 4 distinct vascular territories: the anterior, lateral, posterior, and posterolateral territory. The anterior territory is supplied by the supraorbital and supratrochlear arteries. The lateral territory is the largest of the territories and is supplied by the superficial temporal artery. The posterior territory is divided by the nuchal line into a cephalad and caudal portion. The cephalad area is supplied by the occipital arteries, and the caudal area is supplied by perforating branches from the trapezius and splenius capitis muscles. The posterolateral territory is the smallest territory and is supplied by the posterior auricular artery.[9]

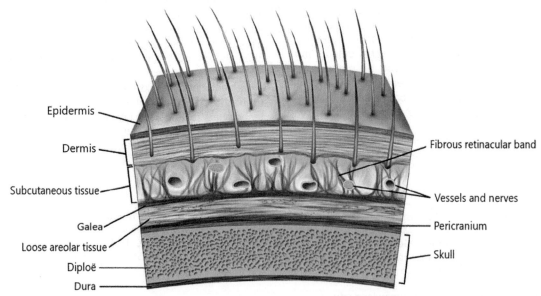

Fig. 1. Soft tissue anatomy of the scalp. (*From* Seline PC, Siegle RJ. Scalp reconstruction. Dermatol Clin. 2005 Jan;23(1):13-21; with permission.)

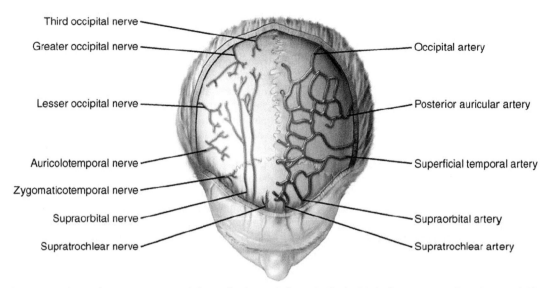

Third occipital nerve
Greater occipital nerve
Lesser occipital nerve
Auriculotemporal nerve
Zygomaticotemporal nerve
Supraorbital nerve
Supratrochlear nerve

Occipital artery
Posterior auricular artery
Superficial temporal artery
Supraorbital artery
Supratrochlear artery

Fig. 2. Vascular and nerve anatomy of the scalp. (*From* Seline PC, Siegle RJ. Scalp reconstruction. Dermatol Clin. 2005 Jan;23(1):13-21; with permission.)

Nerve Anatomy

The sensory innervation of the scalp also has a centripetal distribution and is located within the subcutaneous layer (see **Fig. 2**). The sensation in the anterior and lateral scalp is provided by branches of the trigeminal nerve (supraorbital, zygomaticotemporal, and auriculotemporal nerves). Posteriorly, sensation is provided by branches of the second and third cervical spinal nerves (greater occipital, lesser occipital, and third occipital nerves).[8,9]

Aesthetic Units

Although there are defined anatomic areas of the scalp, which are the occipital, vertex, parietal, and temporal areas, the distribution of hair-bearing scalp is highly variable within the population despite the consistent underlying soft tissue layers especially among men. Despite the variable areas of hair distribution, the scalp is considered to be a singular aesthetic unit. However, when planning for scalp reconstruction, the scalp should be differentiated into the hair-bearing scalp and the non–hair-bearing scalp to optimize aesthetic outcomes.

RECONSTRUCTION PRINCIPLES
Tissue Selection

The goal of soft tissue reconstruction is to provide coverage that is similar in appearance and function, which is encapsulated by the adage: "replace like with like." Thus, the scalp would be the ideal tissue for reconstructing its own defects.

However, the scalp is limited by the distinct set of tissue layers, relative immobility, and the hair-bearing pattern of the area. For these reasons, reconstructing large defects by using the surrounding scalp is often not possible, especially in a single procedure. If nonscalp soft tissues are used for reconstruction, then this may in turn lead to alopecic areas and/or distortion of the normal hairline. Although there may be competing desires from the patient to focus on the aesthetic outcome during their initial reconstruction, the immediate goal should be to provide adequate durable coverage first. Aesthetic outcomes to restore normalcy are important but may only be achieved in staged procedures such as hair transplantation or tissue expansion.[10–13]

Wound Characteristics and Cause

The underlying cause and characteristics of the scalp wound will help guide the reconstruction strategy. The wound evaluation should include the location, size, and depth (ie, involving pericranium, calvarium, dura, etc.) and what adjacent structures may be involved (eg, hairline, eyebrows, etc.). In addition, the quality of the surrounding tissue should also be evaluated. Generally, small- to medium-sized shallow defects with an intact calvarium that have not been previously irradiated, operated on, or are chronically infected are amenable to local flaps. Larger, deeper defects with the presence of these factors are more prone to wound complications and would be better served with vascularized pedicled flaps or free-flap reconstructions.[2,14]

Patient Preference/Goals

Ultimately the reconstruction plan will depend on patient's reconstructive needs, preferences, and comorbidities. In counseling the patient, all of these factors should be taken into account and guide the conversation about different options. For example, reconstruction for a patient undergoing a palliative tumor resection will differ from a young healthy trauma patient with an otherwise disfiguring scalp defect. As it is with the rest of medicine, patient care must be individualized and tailored to each patient's needs and circumstances.

RECONSTRUCTION TECHNIQUES
Primary Closure

The preferred and simplest technique in wound management is primary closure: its simplicity and the approximation of similar tissues will achieve the most natural aesthetic results. Specifically, primary closure in the scalp allows the approximation of hair-bearing areas to minimize irregular alopecic areas and allow for restoration of normal anatomy.[15] However, primary closure is often possible in defects smaller than 3 cm and in tissues that have not been chronically infected, operated on, or have had previous radiation therapy, and often wide undermining is necessary.[15–18] Traumatic scalp lacerations are excellent situations in which primary closure can be pursued. Avulsions without significant tissue loss are also candidates for primary closure after debridement of devitalized tissues due to the complex collateralized vascular system of the scalp. Defects resulting from oncologic resection and/or radiation are generally suboptimal candidates for primary closure, given the larger size and surrounding fibrosis.

Approximating the fibrous galea layer helps with offsetting the tension superficially and limits postoperative alopecia.[18–20] If the galea mobilization is not adequate despite wide undermining, galeal-releasing incisions can be performed perpendicular to the line of wound tension. However, caution must be used so as not to cause iatrogenic injury to the vasculature that lies directly superficial to the galea.[15,18] If the galea is violated, then closure should be performed in layers when possible.

Delayed primary closure is possible with the use of continuous external tissue expanders such as DermaClose (SYNOVIS Micro Companies Alliance, Birmingham, AL). The device, which is applied directly onto the scalp, expands the skin on the subcutaneous planes around the wound in the span of 1 to 2 weeks until the edges are brought close enough together for primary closure (**Fig. 3**).

Secondary Intention

Secondary intention is the oldest technique of wound healing, recorded in Mesopotamian clay tablets from 2500 BC.[21] Secondary intention involves an open wound (with healthy, viable tissue base) to heal from the bottom to top by the formation of granulation tissue.[22] It has become an increasingly prevalent option for treatment of large traumatic wounds since the advent of the vacuum-assisted closure (VAC) device.[23] Traditionally, this technique has often been reserved for patients who may be high-risk surgical candidates or patients with grossly contaminated wounds that are at high risk of infection[24,25]; however, secondary

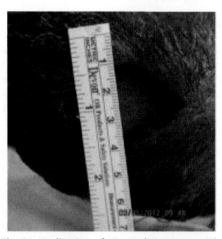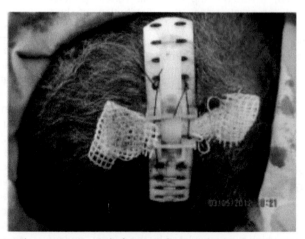

Fig. 3. Application of external tissue expander—TopClosure Tension Relief System (IVT Medical Ltd., Ra'anana, Israel)—on a scalp wound. (*From* Katzengold R, Topaz M, Gefen A. Tissue loads applied by a novel medical device for closing large wounds. J Tissue Viability. 2016 Feb;25(1):32-40; with permission.)

intention offers certain advantages over other methods of wound closure—minimal to no additional incisions or operative procedures, no additional anesthesia, no need for tissue harvest from a donor site, and reliable wound healing in a properly managed wound.[26]

Although the healing process may take weeks to months, the overall success rate has been found to be greater than 80% among a variety of postsurgical wounds.[22] Secondary intention can be used anywhere on the scalp and has been shown to be an effective means of wound healing with an added benefit of better postoperative tumor surveillance in the oncologic resection population.[14,27–29] The healed area will be alopecic; however, because of wound contraction the size of the alopecic area will be smaller.[30] When discussing healing by secondary intention with patients, additional considerations should also be given to the physical and psychological ramifications of this technique, particularly among young patients for whom the open wound is more debilitating and who are more prone to thickened scars due to less skin laxity.[26,31]

Skin Grafts

Skin grafts are a useful reconstructive option for certain scalp defects. In contrast to secondary intention, skin grafts are an expedient and simple method that forgoes the need for long-term wound care at the expense of skin graft harvesting and operative risks. In lesions that are too large for primary closure, skin grafts serve as either a definitive or a temporary measure provided there is an adequate wound bed.[15,32] However, split-thickness skin grafts often result in suboptimal cosmetic results due to differences in pigmentation, texture, and thickness from the surrounding

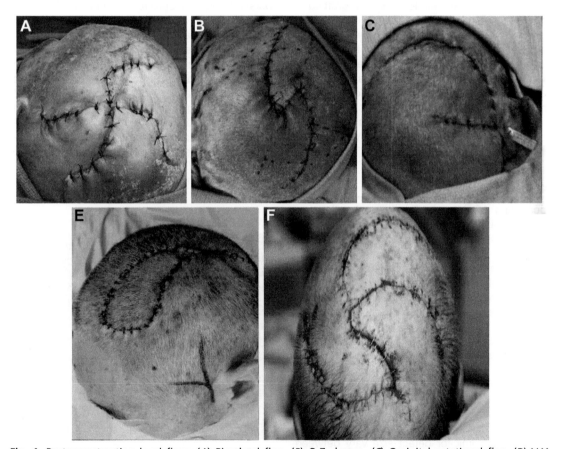

Fig. 4. Postreconstruction local flaps. (*A*) Pinwheel flap. (*B*) O-Z closure. (*C*) Occipital rotational flap. (*D*) V-Y advancement flap. (*E*) Orticochea flap. (*From* [(*A, B, and C*] Sittitavornwong S, Morlandt AB. Reconstruction of the scalp, calvarium, and frontal sinus. Oral Maxillofac Surg Clin North Am. 2013 May;25(2):105-29; with permission; [*D*] Onishi K, Maruyama Y, Hayashi A, Inami K. Repair of scalp defect using a superficial temporal fascia pedicle VY advancement scalp flap. Br J Plast Surg. 2005 Jul;58(5):676-80; with permission; and [*E*] Badhey A, Kadakia S, Abraham MT, Rasamny JK, Moscatello A. Multiflap closure of scalp defects: Revisiting the orticochea flap for scalp reconstruction. Am J Otolaryngol. 2016 Sep-Oct;37(5):466-9; with permission.)

tissues. The grafted surface is usually shiny, immobile, prone to ulceration, and alopecic.[15,17] For this reason, parietal, temporal, and occipital wound sites are more amenable to skin grafting, as these areas are better camouflaged by surrounding hair.[20] In theory, full-thickness skin grafts are more akin to the appearance and texture of normal skin and offer better protection from trauma and radiation with reduced hypopigmentation and secondary contraction.[17,33]

A major limiting factor in skin grafting is the availability of vascularized healing bed. Exposed muscle (eg, temporalis) provides a healthy foundation, and the pericranium alone is also sufficient for graft incorporation. In cases where the pericranium is absent, particularly in oncologic resections, the surgeon can create a healing bed by drilling into or removing most of the calvarial cortex to expose the bleeding diploic space and allow for the formation of granulation tissue (usually with series of VAC dressing changes) for delayed grafting.[18] The use of commercially available regenerative medicine products (eg, collagen/chondroitin matrix, amniotic allograft membrane, fetal bovine dermal/urinary bladder matrix, etc.) have provided more treatment options for the reconstructive surgeons for wound healing/preparation for skin grafting.[34] Skin grafting should be avoided in radiated areas or where radiation is planned, as successful skin grafting requires well-vascularized wound surface.[35,36]

Local Flaps

Local flaps provide excellent reconstruction options for wounds not amenable to primary closure. They have similar texture, appearance, and ability to bear hair, which in turn helps optimize aesthetic results. When evaluating for local flaps, several key factors must be considered to properly tailor the flap to the patient's needs. These factors can be broadly categorized into defect, patient, and flap factors.

Defect factors include location and wound characteristics such as size, exposed structures, cause, and prior radiation treatment.[37,38] Local flap reconstruction in large defects, which is often described as an area greater than 50 cm², have been associated with significantly higher risk of flap-related complications; however, the suggested upper limit for defect size vary between studies.[39,40] In addition, Steiner and colleagues reported that there is an increased likelihood that concomitant skin grafting will be necessary to cover the donor defect, as the size of the defect grows beyond 39.2 cm².[41] Other factors that would make local flap reconstruction a suboptimal

choice would be the presence of bony defects, previous surgical interventions or radiation therapy, and/or plans for adjuvant radiation.[2] Reconstructive surgeons should be an integral part of multidisciplinary discussions for patients undergoing oncologic resection because the reconstructive options may need to be tailored based on plans for adjuvant chemotherapy or radiation.

Patient factors to be considered are health/functional status to determine the operative candidacy, skin quality, and smoking status. Irradiated tissues or chronically scarred tissues are suboptimal for local flap reconstruction, as they confer a high risk of flap complications, in which case free-flap reconstruction should be pursued. In addition, older patients may have a higher chance of success due to skin loosening over time, which would provide more laxity for local flaps. Smokers are at increased risk for complications when undergoing scalp reconstruction, thus tobacco cessation should be pursued before elective reconstruction.[39,42]

Flap factors to be considered are the vascular supply for the flap. Given the extensive collateralized vasculature of the scalp, local flaps usually do not have significant perfusion issues and often do not need to be constructed based on a specific named artery. Larger flaps can be designed based on the advantages of an axial-based perfusion. In small series, local scalp flaps created with a named artery via preoperative ultrasound identification have demonstrated favorable aesthetic contouring and hairline formation.[43] Local flap reconstruction techniques in scalp defects use

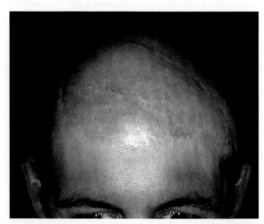

Fig. 5. Final postoperative result after scalp dermatofibrosarcoma protuberans resection with latissimus dorsi free flap and split-thickness skin graft reconstruction. (*From* Shah JP, Patel SG, Singh B et al. Chapter 3: Scalp and Skin. In: Shah JP, Patel SG, Singh B et al, eds. Jatin Shah's Head and Neck Surgery and Oncology. 5th ed. Elsevier; 2020: 27-28.)

the principles of advancement, transposition, and rotation. Advancement and transposition techniques are limited by the flexibility of the galea and the thick poorly distensible nature of the scalp skin. Rotational flaps are well suited for scalp reconstruction; however, longer flap lengths are typically required to compensate for the curvature of the skull.[15,44] Several well-described local flap techniques make use of either one or more of these principles such as the O-Z closure, V-Y advancement flap, Juri flaps, Orticochea flaps, and the pinwheel technique (**Fig. 4**).[33,43–46] Choice of technique will ultimately vary by patient and surgeon preference, but the underlying principles will remain the same: provide safe durable coverage with the best aesthetic result.

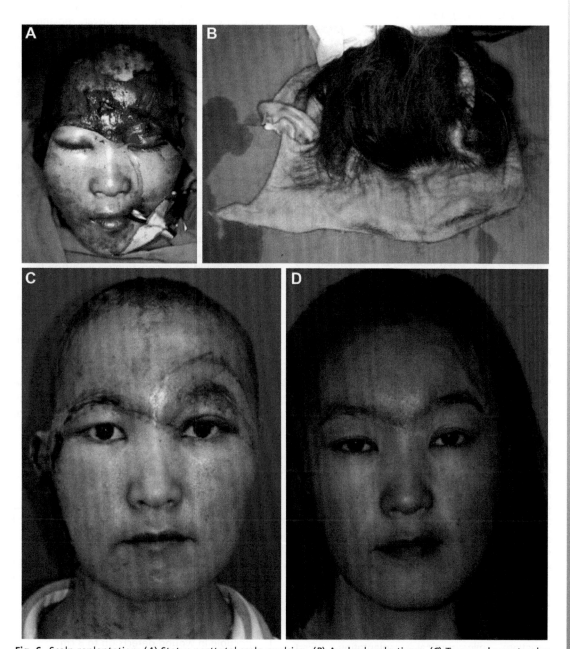

Fig. 6. Scalp replantation: (*A*) Status posttotal scalp avulsion. (*B*) Avulsed scalp tissue. (*C*) Two weeks postreplantation. (*D*) Two years postreplantation. (*From* Kim JT, Kim YH, Yang EZ, Kim JB. Total scalp replantation–salvage following prolonged ischaemia with poor prognostic factors. J Plast Reconstr Aesthet Surg. 2010 Nov;63(11):1917-20.)

Free Flaps

Free tissue transfers are the optimal reconstructive option for wounds that are too large for local flaps, wounds with associated calvarial defects, clinical scenarios where local flap or other reconstruction methods are not feasible or have failed, and/or for patients who received neoadjuvant or will undergo adjuvant radiotherapy. Work-horse flaps for scalp reconstruction include muscle flaps such as the latissimus dorsi (LD), rectus abdominis (RA), and serratus anterior. Skin can be incorporated (ie, myocutaneous) in LD and RA flaps (**Fig. 5**). Fasciocutaneous flaps such as anterolateral thigh (ALT) flaps and radial forearm flaps also provide excellent coverage. ALT flaps can include vastus lateralis muscle if the scalp defect requires bulk to obliterate any dead space.[47–49] The greater omental flap, which is a large peritoneal fold, can cover a very large scalp defect. This flap consists of well-vascularized connective tissue, fat, and lymphatics and is well suited in the setting of contamination and hardware usage. Because harvesting requires laparotomy (or laparoscopy) and there are other available flap options, this flap is used infrequently.[49] When selecting between fasciocutaneous versus muscle flaps, various similar algorithms have been created, and ultimately the decision hinges on the presence of a significant dead space and/or contour abnormality secondary to a calvarial defect.[2,48] Fasciocutaneous flaps are often used when there is no significant dead space or bony defect. Anterolateral thigh flaps in particular have become popular due to the low donor-site morbidity, long pedicle length, adjustable thickness, and large skin paddle.[48] Their use in wounds with calvarial defects have also been described where the well-vascularized fascia has been used to reconstruct dural defects.[48,50,51] Muscle flaps are used when there is a significant dead space, and the latissimus dorsi has been a popular choice due to the ability to cover a large surface area while contouring adequately to the calvarium; however, the rectus abdominis muscle flap has demonstrated excellent results as well.[40,48] The disadvantages of free-flap reconstruction is the need for prolonged operative time, potential for flap complications/failure, and donor-site morbidity.

Replantation

Although total scalp avulsions are a rare event, these injuries allow for a unique method of reconstruction: microsurgical replantation. First described by Miller in 1976, replantation of a viable traumatically avulsed scalp would be the ideal reconstruction choice in these situations.[52] Given the rarity, there is a paucity of literature regarding standardized technique and outcomes beyond case series and reviews. With respect to scalp viability and ischemia time, case reports have shown that the scalp has been able to endure up to 17 and 24 hours of warm and cold ischemia time, respectively, and still be successfully replanted (**Fig. 6**).[53,54] As mentioned previously, the scalp is a richly vascularized area, and thus successful replantation can be performed with a single artery and vein.[4,55] However, replantation failure is frequently reported to be secondary to venous congestion, and thus multiple venous anastomoses should be considered.[56] Also, multiple anastomoses should be considered in instances where the avulsed scalp may be fragmented.

SUMMARY

Soft tissue wounds in the scalp are a common occurrence after trauma or resection of a malignancy. The reconstructive surgeon should strive to use the simplest reconstructive technique while optimizing aesthetic outcomes. In general, defects that are large, infected, previously irradiated (or require postoperative radiation), or have calvarial defects should be reconstructed with free tissue transfer. Smaller defects greater than 3 cm that are not amenable to primary closure may be treated with techniques that can be as simple as allowing for granulation or as complex as local flap reconstruction depending on patient health status, desires, and aesthetic considerations. Total scalp avulsions should be addressed with microsurgical replantation whenever feasible. The reconstructive surgeon should be well versed in various reconstructive options in order to optimize patient care and outcomes.

CLINICS CARE POINTS

- The technique used for scalp reconstruction should be selected based on wound characteristics/cause, patient health status, aesthetic considerations, and patient preferences.
- Increased tension on the reconstructed incision increases the risk of alopecia.
- Primary closure should be attempted when possible in wound defects up to 3 cm.
- To achieve more laxity for closure, galeal-releasing incisions or galeal mobilization via

undermining of the loose areolar tissue layer can be performed.

- Continuous external tissue expanders can aid in achieving delayed primary closure.
- Reconstructive surgeons should be an integral part in multidisciplinary discussions for ablative oncologic procedures.
- The pericranium can serve as an adequate tissue bed for skin grafts.
- Given the extensive vascular network of the scalp, local flaps do not need to be constructed based on a specific named artery.
- Microvascular free tissue transfer should be considered in wounds that are large, chronically infected, have been radiated, or require adjuvant radiation or with calvarial defects.
- Fasciocutaneous free flaps may be used in wounds with no significant dead space or bony defect.
- When microsurgical replantation of a total scalp avulsion is performed, multiple venous anastomoses may be required, and multiple arterial anastomoses should be considered based on tissue fragmentation.

DISCLOSURE

The authors have nothing to disclose.

REFERENCES

1. Ochs M, Chung W, Powers D. Trauma Surgery. J Oral Maxillofac Surg 2017;75(8S):e151–94.
2. Steiner D, Horch RE, Eyüpoglu I, et al. Reconstruction of composite defects of the scalp and neurocranium-a treatment algorithm from local flaps to combined AV loop free flap reconstruction. World J Surg Oncol 2018;16(1):217.
3. Fijałkowska M, Antoszewski B. Complications after scalp suturing posttraumatic avulsion. J Craniofac Surg 2018;29(7):e670–2.
4. Plant MA, Fialkov J. Total scalp avulsion with microvascular reanastomosis: a case report and literature review. Can J Plast Surg 2010;18:112–5.
5. Golpanian S, Kassira W, Habal MB, et al. Treatment options for exposed calvarium due to trauma and burns. J Craniofac Surg 2017;28(2):318–24.
6. Pruzinsky T. Social and psychological effects of major craniofacial deformity. Cleft Palate Craniofac J 1992;29(6):578–84 [discussion: 570].
7. Strayer LM. Augustin Belloste and the treatment of avulsion of the scalp. N Engl J Med 1939;220(22):901.
8. Seery GE. Surgical anatomy of the scalp. Dermatol Surg 2002;28(7):581–7.
9. Leedy JE, Janis JE, Rohrich RJ. Reconstruction of acquired scalp defects: an algorithmic approach. Plast Reconstr Surg 2005;116(4):54e–72e.
10. Yoo H, Moh J, Park JU. Treatment of Postsurgical Scalp Scar Deformity Using Follicular Unit Hair Transplantation. Biomed Res Int 2019;2019:3423657.
11. Jung S, Oh SJ, Hoon Koh S. Hair follicle transplantation on scar tissue. J Craniofac Surg 2013;24(4):1239–41.
12. Barrera A. The use of micrografts and minigrafts for the correction of the postrhytidectomy lost sideburn. Plast Reconstr Surg 1998;102(6):2237–40.
13. Manders EK, Graham WP 3rd, Schenden MJ, et al. Skin expansion to eliminate large scalp defects. Ann Plast Surg 1984;12(4):305–12.
14. Janus JR, Peck BW, Tombers NM, et al. Complications after oncologic scalp reconstruction: a 139-patient series and treatment algorithm. Laryngoscope 2015;125(3):582–8.
15. Earnest LM, Byrne PJ. Scalp reconstruction. Facial Plast Surg Clin North Am 2005;13(2):345–53, vii.
16. Mehrara BJ, Disa JJ, Pusic A. Scalp reconstruction. J Surg Oncol 2006;94(6):504–8.
17. Seitz IA, Gottlieb LJ. Reconstruction of scalp and forehead defects. Clin Plast Surg 2009;36(3):355–77.
18. Desai SC, Sand JP, Sharon JD, et al. Scalp reconstruction: an algorithmic approach and systematic review. JAMA Facial Plast Surg 2015;17(1):56–66.
19. Malone CH, McLaughlin JM, Ross LS, et al. Progressive Tightening of Pulley Sutures for Primary Repair of Large Scalp Wounds. Plast Reconstr Surg Glob Open 2017;5(12):e1592.
20. Seline PC, Siegle RJ. Scalp reconstruction. Dermatol Clin 2005;23(1):13–21, v.
21. Forrest RD. Early history of wound treatment. J R Soc Med 1982;75(3):198–205.
22. Chetter IC, Oswald AV, McGinnis E, et al. Patients with surgical wounds healing by secondary intention: A prospective, cohort study. Int J Nurs Stud 2019;89:62–71.
23. Parrett BM, Matros E, Pribaz JJ, et al. Lower extremity trauma: trends in the management of soft-tissue reconstruction of open tibia-fibula fractures. Plast Reconstr Surg 2006;117(4):1315–22 [discussion: 1323–4].
24. Manthey DE, Nicks BA. Penetrating trauma to the extremity. J Emerg Med 2008;34(2):187–93.
25. O'Connor J, Kells A, Henry S, et al. Vacuum-assisted closure for the treatment of complex chest wounds. Ann Thorac Surg 2005;79(4):1196–200.
26. Goldwyn RM, Rueckert F. The value of healing by secondary intention for sizeable defects of the face. Arch Surg 1977;112(3):285–92.
27. Hoffman JF. Management of scalp defects. Otolaryngol Clin North Am 2001;34(3):571–82.

28. Konofaos P, Kashyap A, Wallace RD. Total scalp reconstruction following a dog bite in a pediatric patient. J Craniofac Surg 2014;25(4):1362–4.

29. Moreno-Arias GA, Izento-Menezes CM, Carrasco MA, et al. Second intention healing after Mohs micrographic surgery. J Eur Acad Dermatol Venereol 2000;14(3):159–65.

30. Becker GD, Adams LA, Levin BC. Secondary intention healing of exposed scalp and forehead bone after Mohs surgery. Otolaryngol Head Neck Surg 1999;121(6):751–4.

31. McCaughan D, Sheard L, Cullum N, et al. Patients' perceptions and experiences of living with a surgical wound healing by secondary intention: A qualitative study. Int J Nurs Stud 2018;77:29–38.

32. Iblher N, Ziegler MC, Penna V, et al. An algorithm for oncologic scalp reconstruction. Plast Reconstr Surg 2010;126(2):450–9 [Erratum in: Plast Reconstr Surg. 2010;126(3):1132].

33. Sittitavornwong S, Morlandt AB. Reconstruction of the scalp, calvarium, and frontal sinus. Oral Maxillofac Surg Clin North Am 2013;25(2):105–29.

34. Khan MA, Ali SN, Farid M, et al. Use of dermal regeneration template (Integra) for reconstruction of full-thickness complex oncologic scalp defects. J Craniofac Surg 2010;21(3):905–9.

35. Tadjalli HE, Evans GR, Gürlek A, et al. Skin graft survival after external beam irradiation. Plast Reconstr Surg 1999;103(7):1902–8.

36. Lawrence WT, Zabell A, McDonald HD. The tolerance of skin grafts to postoperative radiation therapy in patients with soft-tissue sarcoma. Ann Plast Surg 1986;16(3):204–10.

37. Oh SJ, Lee J, Cha J, et al. Free-flap reconstruction of the scalp: donor selection and outcome. J Craniofac Surg 2011;22(3):974–7.

38. Ludolph I, Lehnhardt M, Arkudas A, et al. Plastic reconstructive microsurgery in the elderly patient - Consensus statement of the German Speaking Working Group for Microsurgery of the Peripheral Nerves and Vessels. Handchir Mikrochir Plast Chir 2018;50(2):118–25 [in German].

39. Shonka DC Jr, Potash AE, Jameson MJ, et al. Successful reconstruction of scalp and skull defects: lessons learned from a large series. Laryngoscope 2011;121(11):2305–12.

40. ASh Ooi, Kanapathy M, Ong YS, et al. Optimising Aesthetic Reconstruction of Scalp Soft Tissue by an Algorithm Based on Defect Size and Location. Ann Acad Med Singap 2015;44(11):535–41.

41. Steiner D, Hubertus A, Arkudas A, et al. Scalp reconstruction: A 10-year retrospective study. J Craniomaxillofac Surg 2017;45(2):319–24.

42. Wang CY, Dudzinski J, Nguyen D, et al. Association of Smoking and Other Factors With the Outcome of Mohs Reconstruction Using Flaps or Grafts. JAMA Facial Plast Surg 2019;21(5):407–13.

43. Shen H, Dai X, Chen J, et al. Modified Unilateral Pedicled V-Y Advancement Flap for Scalp Defect Repair. J Craniofac Surg 2018;29(3):608–13.

44. Costa DJ, Walen S, Varvares M, et al. Scalp Rotation Flap for Reconstruction of Complex Soft Tissue Defects. J Neurol Surg B Skull Base 2016;77(1):32–7.

45. Chou PY, Lin CH, Hsu CC, et al. Salvage of postcranioplasty implant exposure using free tissue transfer. Head Neck 2017;39(8):1655–61.

46. Badhey A, Kadakia S, Abraham MT, et al. Multiflap closure of scalp defects: Revisiting the orticochea flap for scalp reconstruction. Am J Otolaryngol 2016;37(5):466–9.

47. Beasley NJ, Gilbert RW, Gullane PJ, et al. Scalp and forehead reconstruction using free revascularized tissue transfer. Arch Facial Plast Surg 2004;6(1):16–20.

48. Chang KP, Lai CH, Chang CH, et al. Free flap options for reconstruction of complicated scalp and calvarial defects: report of a series of cases and literature review. Microsurgery 2010;30(1):13–8.

49. Hultman CS, Carlson GW, Losken A, et al. Utility of the omentum in the reconstruction of complex extraperitoneal wounds and defects: donor-site complications in 135 patients from 1975 to 2000. Ann Surg 2002;235(6):782–95.

50. Ozkan O, Coskunfirat OK, Ozgentas HE, et al. Rationale for reconstruction of large scalp defects using the anterolateral thigh flap: Structural and aesthetic outcomes. J Reconstr Microsurg 2005;21:539–45.

51. Heller F, Hsu CM, Chuang CC, et al. Anterolateral thigh fasciocutaneous flap for simultaneous reconstruction of refractory scalp and dural defects. Report of two cases. J Neurosurg 2004;100:1094–7.

52. Miller GD, Anstee EJ, Snell JA. Successful replantation of an avulsed scalp by microvascular anastomoses. Plast Reconstr Surg 1976;58(2):133–6.

53. Juri J, Irigaray A, Zeaiter C. Reimplantation of scalp. Ann Plast Surg 1990;24(4):354–61.

54. Sirimaharaj W, Boonpadhanapong T. Scalp replantation: a case report of long ischemic time. J Med Assoc Thai 2001;84(11):1629–34.

55. Nahai F, Hurteau J, Vasconez LO. Replantation of an entire scalp and ear by microvascular anastomoses of only 1 artery and 1 vein. Br J Plast Surg 1978;31(4):339–42.

56. Kim EK, Kim SC. Total scalp replantation salvaged by changing the recipient vein. J Craniofac Surg 2012;23(5):1428–9.

Management of Laryngeal Trauma

Nadir Elias, DMD[a], James Thomas, MD[b], Allen Cheng, MD, DDS[c],*

KEYWORDS

- Laryngeal trauma • Laryngotracheal injury • Laryngofissure

KEY POINTS

- The key step in treatment of any laryngeal injury is the establishment of a secure airway.
- Early intervention (within 24–48 hours) is an important factor for improved patient outcomes (functional speech, swallowing, and airway patency).
- An awake tracheostomy is the airway of choice with grade II or higher laryngeal injuries.

INTRODUCTION

The larynx is a complex anatomic structure and a properly functioning larynx is essential for breathing, voice, and swallowing. Injuries to the larynx and trachea can result in significant and potentially fatal consequences. Laryngeal trauma is often associated with other injuries, including intracranial injuries (17%), penetrating neck injuries (18%), cervical spine fractures (13%), and facial fractures (9%).[1] Laryngeal injuries are rare, occurring in only 1 of 5000 to 137,000 emergency room visits[1–3] and among only 1 in 445 patients with severe injuries.[4] Because of this, even surgeons with a great deal of experience in managing maxillofacial trauma have limited exposure to management of laryngeal and tracheal injury. This article discusses the evaluation, diagnosis, and management of patients with laryngeal and tracheal injury.

CLASSIFICATION OF LARYNGEAL INJURIES

Several classification systems have been described to assist in developing an algorithmic approach to managing these difficult and rare injuries. These classification systems have been based on mode of injury, types of tissues involved in the injury, anatomic locations of injury, and severity of the injury. Modes of injury have been divided into blunt and penetrating injuries.

Whereas blunt injuries have been described as being associated with greater length of hospitalization,[5] our experience has been that penetrating airway injuries, often associated with ballistic wounds, are much more likely to be associated with greater endolaryngeal disruption. The types of tissues involved have been divided into hard and soft tissue injuries. Locations of injuries have been classified as injuries that affect the supraglottic larynx, the glottis, and subglottic larynx.

Lynch[5] was the first to classify traumatic injuries based on location. In 1969, Nahum[6] described laryngeal injuries based on injury location and likelihood of recovery with and without intervention. In 1980, Schaefer and colleagues developed what has become the most popular classification system to assess the severity of such injuries.[7] This classification describes laryngeal injuries on a scale of I-IV. Schaefer's classification was later modified by Fuhrman and colleagues[8] to include laryngotracheal separation (**Table 1**) and again by Verschueren and colleagues[4] in 2006 to include the use of computed tomography (CT) imaging in staging (**Table 2**). In this article, the discussion of the initial evaluation and management of a patient with laryngeal trauma is within the framework of the Legacy Emanuel Classification, as outlined by the algorithm in **Fig. 1**. However, the principles are generalizable and can be applied to whichever system the reader finds most helpful in their practice.

[a] Advanced Craniomaxillofacial and Trauma Surgery, Legacy Emanuel Medical Center, 1849 NW Kearney Street, Suite 300, Portland, OR 97209, USA; [b] Private Practice, Voicedoctor.net, 909 NW 18th Avenue, Portland, OR 97209, USA; [c] Oral/Head and Neck Oncology, Legacy Good Samaritan Cancer Center, Portland, OR, USA
* Corresponding author. 1849 Northwest Kearney, Suite 300, Portland, OR 97209.
E-mail address: chenga@head-neck.com

Oral Maxillofacial Surg Clin N Am 33 (2021) 417–427
https://doi.org/10.1016/j.coms.2021.04.007
1042-3699/21/© 2021 Elsevier Inc. All rights reserved.

Table 1
Fuhrman-Schaefer classification of laryngeal injuries

Stage	Injury
I	Minor laryngeal hematoma, edema, laceration; no detectable fracture
II	Edema, hematoma, mucosal disruption with no exposed cartilage, nondisplaced fractures
III	Significant edema, noted mucosal disruption, exposed cartilage with or without cord immobility, displaced fractures
IV	Significant edema, noted mucosal disruption, exposed cartilage with or without cord immobility, displaced fractures with 2 or more fracture lines, skeletal instability/anterior commissure trauma
V	Complete laryngotracheal separation

INITIAL EVALUATION AND INITIAL MANAGEMENT

The initial evaluation of a patient suspected of having laryngeal or tracheal injury, as with any trauma, begins with the primary survey as outlined in Advanced Trauma Life Support algorithms. Because the larynx and trachea are critical components of the airway, prompt identification and management of these injuries are prioritized. This

Table 2
Legacy Emanuel Medical Center laryngeal injury classification

Stage	Diagnostic Findings	Management
I	Minor airway symptoms ± Voice changes No fractures Small lacerations	Observation Humidified air Head of bed elevation
II	Airway compromise Nondisplaced fractures No cartilage exposure Voice changes ± Subcutaneous emphysema	Immediate awake tracheostomy if airway not already secured in the field Humidified air Head of bed elevation ± ORIF
III	Airway compromise Edema Mucosal lacerations Palpable laryngeal fractures Exposed cartilage Subcutaneous emphysemas Voice changes	Immediate awake tracheostomy if airway not already secured in the field Direct laryngoscopy Exploration and ORIF
IV	Airway compromise Mucosal lacerations Exposed cartilage Palpable displaced laryngeal fractures with skeletal instability Subcutaneous emphysemas Voice changes	Immediate awake tracheostomy if airway not already secured in the field Direct laryngoscopy Exploration/ORIF Consider stenting

Abbreviation: ORIF, open reduction internal fixation.
Adapted from Verschueren DS, Bell RB, Bagheri SC, Dierks EJ, Potter BE. Management of laryngo-tracheal injuries associated with craniomaxillofacial trauma. J Oral Maxillofac Surg. 2006 Feb;64(2):203-14; with permission.

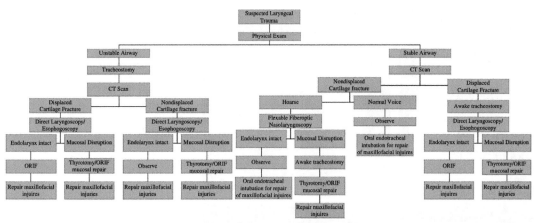

Fig. 1. Protocol for management of laryngotracheal injuries at Legacy Emanuel Hospital and Health Center in Portland, Oregon. ORIF, open reduction internal fixation. (*From* Verschueren DS, Bell RB, Bagheri SC, Dierks EJ, Potter BE. Management of laryngo-tracheal injuries associated with craniomaxillofacial trauma. J Oral Maxillofac Surg. 2006 Feb;64(2):203-14; with permission.)

begins with a quick survey of the injuries. Patients with either blunt or penetrating injury to the neck must be ruled out as having airway injury. The mechanism of the injury should also raise one's suspicion. In a review of laryngeal injuries from 1992 to 2004, high speed motor vehicle accidents were the most common mechanism (49%), followed by sports-related injuries (29%).[4] Certain mechanisms of injury, such as hanging, gunshot wounds, or work-related high-energy injuries to the neck, should obviously generate an elevated level of suspicion.

Stable Versus Unstable Airway

The first essential question is to establish whether the airway is secured and whether the patient is stable. If the patient is stable and protecting their airway, there is time for a more deliberate examination. This is important because occult trachea-laryngeal disturbance can occur with minimal external signs of trauma.

The initial airway physical examination starts with visual inspection for swelling, soft tissue injury overlying the airway, loss of anatomic landmarks in the neck, and signs of troubled breathing. A cursory examination of the patient's voice is performed, noting the presence or absence of stridor and/or dysphonia. Next, use gentle palpation to assess for subcutaneous emphysema and palpable disruption of the hyoid bone, thyroid cartilage, cricoid, and trachea. The most common findings on physical examination include subcutaneous air, hoarseness, tenderness of the anterior neck to palpation, and stridor.[9]

A fiberoptic examination may also be performed if timing allows and other injuries do not take precedence. The fiberoptic examination may help to verify that the patient's airway is stable enough for transfer to the scanner. An awake fiberoptic examination also has the benefit of allowing visualization of the larynx in function. This examination is meant to be performed quickly and efficiently so as to not impede overall trauma management. The evaluating surgeon must keep in mind that traumatized airways that appear stable tend to deteriorate over time because of the onset of edema, expansion of hematomas, and other contributory factors.

The next step is a CT scan of the head and neck, which is done in addition to CT scans of chest, abdomen, and pelvis that are routinely performed as part of the trauma survey (**Fig. 2**). In stable patients with penetrating neck injury, a CT angiogram is also included to evaluate for vascular injury. CT imaging allows for rapid and accurate identification of hard tissue injuries to larynx and trachea and identification of soft tissue air emphysema.[10]

If the airway is not secure and/or is unstable, or the patient is unstable for other reasons, the patient is taken emergently to the operating room where securing the airway followed by stabilization of the patient is the immediate priority. Traditionally, this is via an oral endotracheal intubation. However, if the patient has a known laryngeal or tracheal injury, oral endotracheal intubation can fail, particularly because of false passage or further disruption of the injured airway. Although securing the airway trumps any other priority, in this situation the most ideal airway is a tracheostomy, performed awake with either mask or laryngeal mask airway support, as the situation allows. If endotracheal intubation is the route chosen, a fiberoptic intubation with a pediatric bronchoscope is one of several tools

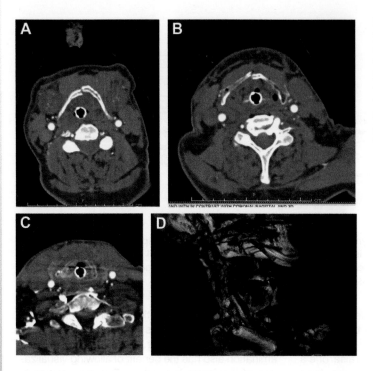

Fig. 2. Axial CT neck images of a 64-year-old male victim of a motorcycle accident with severe multisystem trauma. Injuries included (*A*) hyoid bone fracture, (*B*) a thyroid cartilage fracture, and (*C*) and cricoid cartilage fracture. (*D*) Three-dimensional reconstruction of the CT demonstrating the previously mentioned fractures.

to be considered by the anesthesiologist. In the presence of endolaryngeal lacerations, the primary risk is that of intubating a blind submuco-perichondrial pouch that produces immediate and total airway obstruction. The stat surgical airway that follows not only risks the patient's life but can also worsen the existing laryngotracheal injuries.

Once the airway is secured and the patient is stable, the next step in the evaluation involves physical examination, CT imaging (if not already performed), and panendoscopy. Anatomically, the larynx is subdivided into the supraglottic larynx, glottic larynx, and subglottic larynx, and trachea. Injury can occur at any and all of these levels. Therefore, the examination is performed in such manner where each of these areas are carefully inspected. It is important to remember that, particularly with blunt trauma, disruption of the laryngeal framework can occur without obvious external findings. For example, disruption of the cricoarytenoid joint and shortening of the true vocal cord can occur with blunt trauma and manifest itself with vocal changes, without external signs of injury. If left untreated, the dislocated arytenoid may scar in that position resulting in permanent, more difficult to correct vocal disturbance. It is widely agreed on that early identification and treatment of laryngeal injuries yields superior results, ideally within the first 24 to 48 hours if circumstances allow.

Nondisplaced Versus Displaced Cartilage Fractures

The CT scan answers an essential branch point in our management algorithm, which is whether or not there are displaced fractures of the cartilaginous larynx. The CT scan is especially valuable because it can detect occult fractures missed on examination.[11]

Patients without cartilage fractures or with nondisplaced cartilage fractures are managed in a more conservative manner. Patients with nondisplaced cartilage fractures are carefully assessed for vocal disturbances. Signs of voice changes should prompt a fiberoptic nasopharyngoscopy to assess for endolaryngeal injury. If the patient has already been intubated or has a tracheostomy, a direct laryngoscopy under anesthesia is performed instead. While under anesthesia, a bronchoscopy and esophagoscopy are also performed to assess the full extent of injury.

If no signs of endolaryngeal injury are observed, the patient is observed and receives supportive care. If the laryngeal examination demonstrates mucosal injury, consideration should be given to surgical repair versus serial endoscopic examination. Mucosal lacerations are repaired primarily through a thyrotomy (laryngofissure) approach, or in some cases, endoscopically. Denuded laryngeal cartilage that is not amenable to primary closure is treated with a thyrotomy approach coupled with use of a laryngeal stent or laryngeal keel.[12]

If the CT scan identifies displaced cartilage fractures, these are treated with open reduction and internal fixation. Before this, many such patients benefit from having the airway secured with an awake tracheostomy. This avoids the need for endotracheal intubation, which is challenging and further disrupts the displaced cartilage fractures. Once the airway is secured, direct laryngoscopy is performed to assess for endolaryngeal injury, as discussed previously. Consideration is given to including esophagoscopy and/or bronchoscopy. If there are no signs of endolaryngeal injury, the surgeon may proceed with open reduction and internal fixation of the displaced cartilage segments. If there are signs of significant endolaryngeal injury, repair them via laryngofissure approach followed by open reduction internal fixation of the cartilage fractures.

ANATOMIC CONSIDERATIONS
Epiglottis

The epiglottis, as the superior extent of the supraglottic larynx, connected by ligaments to the hyoid bone and thyroid cartilage, is significantly affected by laryngeal trauma. Hyoid fractures can result in an epiglottic hematoma (**Fig. 3**). An epiglottic

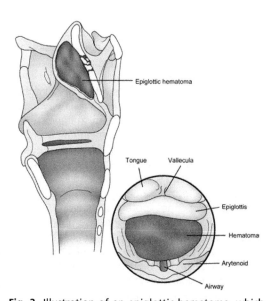

Fig. 3. Illustration of an epiglottic hematoma, which may result from hyoid or thyroid fracture. Note that as the hematoma expands, the airway is at risk for critical obstruction. (*From* Bell RB, Verschueren DS, Dierks EJ. Management of laryngeal trauma. Oral Maxillofac Surg Clin North Am. 2008 Aug;20(3):415-30; with permission.)

hematoma quickly results in stridor, difficulty with speech, and eventually dyspnea and potential airway embarrassment. Partial or complete avulsion of the epiglottis can also occur with severe hyoid and thyroid fractures. This manifests as dysphagia and aspiration.

Hyoid Bone Fractures

Hyoid bone fractures are a result of high-energy impact and, in our Legacy Emanuel series, were often seen in sporting injuries, such as baseball, jet skiing, and martial arts.[4] Such injuries are also seen in suicidal hanging and in attempted manual strangulation. Most hyoid fractures do not require surgical intervention. However, they are usually accompanied by temporary odynophagia. Significantly displaced hyoid fractures are managed by either open reduction and internal fixation of the hyoid bone or partial hyoid resection.

Distortion of the Glottis

Injury to the larynx can result in changes in the anterior-posterior dimension of the vocal cords, the positioning of the vocal cords relative to each other, the mobility of the cords, and soft tissue injury of the cords. Any of these distortions can result in voice changes. Voice changes of volume loss and pitch lowering indicate shortening of the vocal cords. Voice changes of roughness indicate asymmetry of the vocal cords, such as a unilateral change in length or asymmetric swelling.

Displaced fractures of the thyroid cartilage involving the anterior commissure and/or arytenoid dislocation can result in foreshortening of the vocal cords. This is identified on endoscopic examination, confirmed on CT scan, and is a strong indication for open reduction internal fixation (**Fig. 4**).

Mucosal injury involving the vocal cords that remains unrepaired will heal by secondary intention, but such healing can result in synechiae between opposing vocal cords and at the anterior commissure. Careful inspection for such injuries is essential and their presence is an indication for repair.

Cricoid Injury and Cricotracheal/Laryngotracheal Separation

Injury of the subglottic larynx can result in cricoid fractures and/or cricotracheal separation, both of which result in devastating airway obstruction that is difficult to rescue in the field because these generally require an emergent tracheostomy. Patients who are able to be stabilized are often found to have recurrent laryngeal nerve injury.

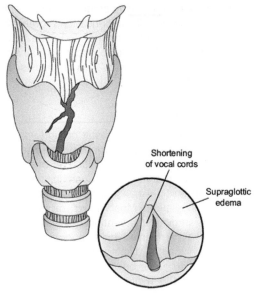

Fig. 4. Fracture of the thyroid cartilage may result in edema, shortening, and possible avulsion of the vocal cords resulting in significant voice changes. (*From* Bell RB, Verschueren DS, Dierks EJ. Management of laryngeal trauma. Oral Maxillofac Surg Clin North Am. 2008 Aug;20(3):415-30; with permission.)

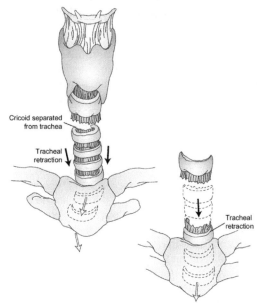

Fig. 5. Complete laryngotracheal separation with tracheal retraction may result in profound airway compromise and death if not treated with immediate airway stabilization in the form a tracheostomy. (*From* Bell RB, Verschueren DS, Dierks EJ. Management of laryngeal trauma. Oral Maxillofac Surg Clin North Am. 2008 Aug;20(3):415-30; with permission.)

If the larynx or cricoid becomes separated from the trachea, the trachea tends to retract inferiorly toward the mediastinum (**Fig. 5**). Reconstruction requires limited circumferential dissection of the trachea to allow placement of bolstering sutures for tension-free approximation of the divided airway.

OPERATIVE TECHNIQUE
Endoscopy

It is beyond the scope of this article to discuss the nuances of performing endoscopic examination of the upper aerodigestive tract. However, we will discuss some pearls related to these techniques.

Flexible nasopharyngoscopy is an efficient, widely available (found on most hospital airway carts), and effective way to examine the airway in an awake or sedated patient. Performing this on an awake patient affords the benefit of being able to visualize the larynx in function, specifically the presence of absence of vocal cord motion. The effective performance of this examination in an awake trauma patient is uniquely challenging. Blood and swelling in the airway or difficulty with topical anesthesia in an agitated patient can make good visualization impossible.

In these cases, performance of an endoscopic examination in an anesthetized patient after the airway has been secured is the other option.

This is ideally performed directly using a laryngoscope, because this can address the collapse of the potential space that occurs when a patient is in a supine position. However, many trauma patients with airway injury are at risk of cervical spine injury and remain on cervical spine precautions that limit neck extension. This difficulty is compounded among patients with classic intubation challenges, such as anterior airways and mandibular hypoplasia. In such instances, we revert back to fiberoptic examination assisted by a videolaryngoscope. A videolaryngoscope is introduced in the traditional fashion, with the tip of the blade placed within the vallecula. This suspends the base of tongue and mandible anteriorly, opening the potential space in the oropharynx, which allows the fiberoptic scope to be more useful.

Examination of the trachea is performed with either a flexible or rigid bronchoscope. In the trauma setting, the flexible bronchoscope is the simplest to use, does not require neck extension, and allows creation of video documentation of the injuries.

Examination of the cervical and thoracic esophagus is performed either with a rigid or flexible esophagoscopy. Rigid esophagoscopy is thought to be more sensitive than flexible esophagoscopy in identifying injuries.[13] It also does not require insufflation to create a potential space for visualization, which runs the risk of causing soft tissue air emphysema in the mediastinum and neck. However, as with laryngoscopy, it is difficult to perform on patients in a cervical collar and those with anatomic limitations. Also, a rigid esophagoscope also runs the risk of further disrupting an injured larynx.

Tracheostomy

The tracheostomy is a routine procedure that is a valuable part of the armamentarium of any surgeon active in trauma. There are also as many ways to perform the procedure as there are surgeons performing it. As such, we focus this discussion not on how to perform a tracheostomy, but modifications for performing a tracheostomy in a patient likely to have laryngeal injury.

Tracheostomy in this setting is often performed before the patient's cervical spine has been cleared. As such, maintaining neck immobilization is paramount. The head is typically stabilized with tape to the bed or operating table while the anterior portion of the cervical collar is removed for access. Additional support to the neck is provided by the anesthesiologist.

As previously mentioned, it is ideal to perform an awake tracheostomy. This requires a concerted effort between the anesthesiologist and surgeon. Although the procedure is described as "awake," it is most optimally performed with some degree of sedation. This is typically a combination of an amnestic with a general anesthetic at a dose that maintains spontaneous respiration. In addition to oxygenation, mask ventilatory support, typically by face mask, is essential. Good local anesthesia is of critical importance. We typically deliver field blocks to the cervical plexus along the anterior border of the sternocleidomastoid muscle on either side and infiltration from the skin down to the trachea.

In the absence of useful overlying lacerations, a horizontal incision is used for the tracheostomy at a level that can be incorporated into an apron incision later for neck exploration, if needed.

Once the trachea is visualized, the tracheotomy should ideally be placed distal to the injury, usually between the third and fourth tracheal rings. Although a cricothyroidotomy is the most expedient in an emergency situation, it does interfere with laryngeal reconstruction and risks limiting cricothyroid mobility in the future (limiting upper vocal range and maximal volume). If a cricothyroidotomy has been previously performed, the airway should be converted to a tracheostomy as soon as it is practical.

Surgical Exposure

If existing lacerations do not provide sufficient exposure, a limited neck exploration may be necessary. A horizontal incision is designed that is made to incorporate the incision of the tracheostomy. The incision is wide enough to explore the lateral neck if necessitated by the nature of the injury. The skin flaps are developed in a suprafascial plane over the strap musculature. The flaps are elevated superiorly to the level of the hyoid bone and inferiorly to the clavicles.

If broader exposure is necessary, the sternocleidomastoid muscles are skeletonized on the medial/deep sides for access to create an outer tunnel. Blunt and sharp dissection are used medial to the carotid sheath allowing lateral retraction to create the inner tunnel. This allows wide access to the larynx, pharynx, and esophagus on either side.

The median raphe is identified and dissection is carried in this plane through the infrahyoid strap muscles. The strap muscles are bluntly dissected and retracted laterally until the thyroid cartilage is visualized (**Fig. 6**).

Endolaryngeal repair and reconstruction is accessed by performing a laryngofissure using a midline thyrotomy, if the exposure has not already been created by the injury. A horizontal incision is made through the cricothyroid membrane. Using a 12 blade, and under the direct visualization, cut from an inferior to superior direction directly between the true vocal cords in the midline. This is important, because detachment or further disruption of the vocal cord at the anterior commissure is difficult to correct. An oscillating saw is used to complete the midline thyrotomy. The two sides of the thyroid cartilage can then be retracted laterally (**Fig. 7**).

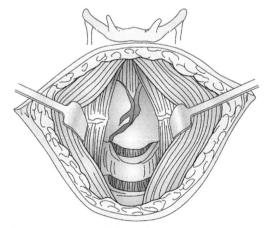

Fig. 6. Retraction of the strap musculature to allow for visualization of the cartilaginous injuries. (*From* Bell RB, Verschueren DS, Dierks EJ. Management of laryngeal trauma. Oral Maxillofac Surg Clin North Am. 2008 Aug;20(3):415-30; with permission.)

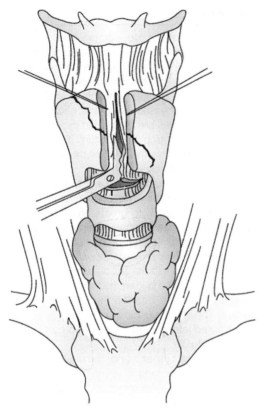

Fig. 7. Midline thyrotomy allows for lateral retraction of the thyroid and cricoid cartilages to allow for visualization of laryngeal and esophageal structures. (*From* Bell RB, Verschueren DS, Dierks EJ. Management of laryngeal trauma. Oral Maxillofac Surg Clin North Am. 2008 Aug;20(3):415-30; with permission.)

Alternatively, for surgeons with greater experience, a simpler method involves starting with a midline thyroidotomy. The oscillating saw is used to make a cut in the midline and the two halves of the thyroid cartilage are gently pulled to 3 to 4 mm apart. Generally, if performed with care this is executed without violating the mucosa and entering the airway. The vocal processes are visually identified as two white spots. They can be divided in the midline and remain attached to their respective thyroid ala. This obviates an incision in the cricothyroid area and allows improved airtight closure.

If the airway is inadvertently entered during thyroid cartilage division, it will nearly always be into the space between the true and false vocal cords, the thinnest area of mucosa. Using an 11 blade, the vocal ligaments are divided. Up-angled scissors can divide the false cords if needed for visualization. One can then leave the inferior mucosa intact for an airtight seal after closure.

If an esophageal injury has been identified, this should be repaired before the endolaryngeal repair.

Endolaryngeal Repair

After the laryngofissure is performed, the supraglottic, glottic, and subglottic larynx is directly visualized. Mucosal lacerations, particularly if there is exposed cartilage, are repaired primarily with resorbable sutures, such as 4–0 and 5–0 chromic gut. Do not debride lacerated mucosa, because this makes primary closure difficult. The arytenoids are inspected. If dislocated, they should be reduced. The vocal cord attachments to the thyroid cartilage are also inspected. If there is detachment, the vocal cords are resuspended using fine nonresorbable suture to the thyroid cartilage at Broyles ligament (**Fig. 8**).

Rarely, there may be avulsion injuries of the mucosa that are not amenable to primary closure. Special consideration is given to these, particularly if there are opposing injuries on the other side. This may result in adhesions that inhibit vocal cord mobility. This is managed using a laryngeal stent or a keel. A laryngeal stent is placed with or without a skin graft (with the underside of the graft facing outward) (**Fig. 9**). The stent is then secured with two nonresorbable sutures. The first suture is passed through skin, thyroid lamina, stent, opposite thyroid lamina, and back out through the skin. The second suture is passed through skin, subglottic trachea, stent, opposite wall of the trachea, and back out through skin. The two sutures are passed through an external silicone button and tied loosely, on either side. The primary advantage of the stent, beyond preventing synechiae and adhesions, is that it provides structural stabilization of the endolarynx circumferentially. By separating denuded areas from each other, it allows for epithelial migration and healing by secondary intention without adhesions. However, it comes at some risk. The stent itself may cause pressure on the endolaryngeal mucosa, creating raw areas that may heal as adhesions once the stent is removed. This may result in stenosis later on.

An alternative to a laryngeal stent is the use of a keel. Similar to a stent, it is a barrier that allows for healing by secondary to intention while preventing adhesions. In contrast to a stent, it does not provide circumferential support of the larynx. This avoids the risk of pressure or rubbing injury to the endolaryngeal mucosa.

The laryngofissure must be meticulously repaired. Fine nonresorbable sutures are used to reconstruct the anterior commissure. Special attention is given to lining up these two landmarks

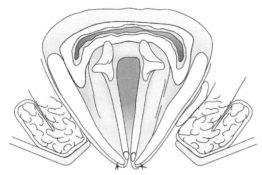

Fig. 8. Resuspension of Broyles ligament to the external perichondrium. (*From* Bell RB, Verschueren DS, Dierks EJ. Management of laryngeal trauma. Oral Maxillofac Surg Clin North Am. 2008 Aug;20(3):415-30; with permission.)

in the same horizontal plane, otherwise the vocal cords do not adduct evenly during function. A suture is passed through the thyroid cartilage and anterior commissure on one side, then through the anterior commissure and thyroid cartilage on the opposite side to line these points up correctly.

The thyroid (and cricoid, if necessary) is then repaired either with suture, wire, or miniplate fixation (**Fig. 10**). When using miniplates, be sure to choose screws that do not penetrate the endolaryngeal mucosa. Resorbable plates and screws have also been used for this indication.

Reconstruction of Cricotracheal Separation

For reconstruction of a complete separation of the trachea from the larynx, the trachea must be sufficiently mobilized. Blunt dissection is used anterior

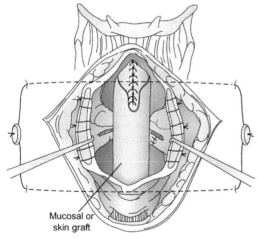

Mucosal or skin graft

Fig. 9. A laryngeal stent can be secured with sutures that extend through the skin, thyroid lamina bilaterally before being tied loosely over skin buttons. (*From* Bell RB, Verschueren DS, Dierks EJ. Management of laryngeal trauma. Oral Maxillofac Surg Clin North Am. 2008 Aug;20(3):415-30; with permission.)

and posterior to the trachea. This can often be done carefully with a finger. Avoid excessive lateral dissection, because this may compromise the vascular supply to the skeletonized trachea. This dissection should be carried inferiorly into the superior mediastinum to allow for sufficient superior traction.

Nonresorbable sutures, such as 2–0 Prolene, are used to reconstruct. These sutures are passed through the cartilage of a tracheal ring at least one or more rings distal the injury. Superiorly, the suture needle is then passed through the cricoid. Be sure to avoid passing through the tracheal mucosa. These sutures are placed 270° around the trachea. Once all the sutures are passed, they are tied down one by one, working from lateral to anterior (**Fig. 11**). It is important to keep the patient's head out of extension, to minimize tension across the closure. As a reminder to the patient, a Grillo stitch, a heavy nonresorbable suture passed from menton to sternum, is placed. This discourages the patient from extending his or her neck and putting excess tension across the repaired trachea.

After the repair is complete, the patient can usually be extubated, assuming other indications for remaining intubated are not present. However, keeping the patient intubated may be prudent, depending on the surgeon's judgment and the patient's clinical status.

Wound Closure

The skin flaps are closed in layers. Special attention must be given to separation of the tracheostomy from the rest of the wound. Deep sutures are placed circumferentially around the tracheostomy to seal it off. Suction drains are placed under the skin flaps to prevent saliva or seroma accumulation or a subcutaneous aerocele. Although some authors advocate for passive drains for fear of promotion of fistula formation, we have not found this to be an issue in our experience.

POSTOPERATIVE CARE
Enteral Feeds

The patient is initially fed by a nasogastric feeding tube because temporary dysphagia is common. Enteral feeds are continued until the patient is able to protect their airway. If permitted by other injuries, a swallow evaluation is initiated by a speech language pathologist as early as the third to fourth postoperative day. If aspiration is present, enteral feeds are continued until this is resolved.

If there was an esophageal injury, we typically postpone initiation of oral feeding for 2 weeks. Before oral feeding, a modified barium swallow and esophogram are performed to assess for leaks.

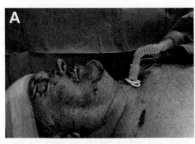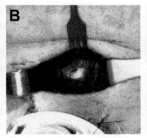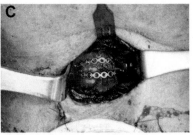

Fig. 10. A 64-year-old male victim whose CT images were presented in **Fig. 4**. Examination of the neck revealed and large submental laceration and edema and ecchymosis extending down to the sternal notch, which raised the suspicion for a laryngeal injury. (*A*) Clinical appearance after initial stabilization with a tracheostomy. (*B*) Intraoperative exposure for repair of the laryngeal injuries. (*C*) Open reduction internal fixation of thyroid and cricoid cartilages.

If leaks are present, enteral feeds are continued for an additional 2 weeks and the study is repeated.

COMPLICATIONS

Several perioperative complications can occur with laryngotracheal injuries including voice changes; bleeding; infection; fistula formation; and, most seriously, loss of airway. However, probably the most substantial and common long-term issue is stenosis of the airway. This can occur in the presence of mucosal injuries that results in adhesions or wound contracture. Circumferential injuries are at the greatest risk. Despite careful mucosal repair and use of stents, stenosis can still occur. This is a chronic and difficult to manage problem. Even with a patent airway, a stenotic airway can result in stridor, dyspnea on mild exertion, constant shortness of breath, and intractable fatigue. Such patients often undergo tracheostomy and subsequently seek tracheal "sleeve" resection.

Initial management of airway stenosis starts with a careful endoscopic examination to identify the

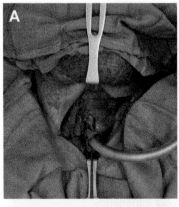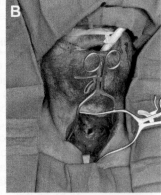
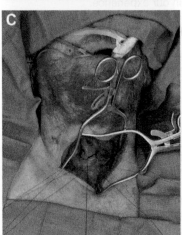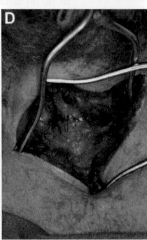

Fig. 11. Patient suffered a work-related injury where a chain saw rebounded off a metal pipe resulting in a penetrating anterior neck injury that led to near complete cricotracheal separation. An emergency medical technician in the field visualized bubbles from his neck wound and was able to intubate his trachea directly and secure his airway. He was immediately taken to Legacy Emanuel Medical Center, directly to the operating room. (*A*) After hemostasis was obtained and panendoscopy performed, the "trach" was converted to an oral endotracheal tube. (*B*) The trachea was mobilized with blunt dissection. (*C*) 2–0 Prolene sutures were used to repair the separation. Note the sutures are passed through a tracheal ring away from the site of injury. (*D*) The patient's neck was placed in slight flexion and the sutures tied down in a parachuting fashion.

location, length, and degree of stenosis. Tracheal stenosis isolated to a few rings is often amenable to serial bronchoscopic partial laser ablations combined with careful dilation. In severe, refractory tracheal stenosis below the second ring, tracheal resection of several rings and primary anastomosis is performed. Stenosis involving the cricoid is generally managed by cricoid split with interpositional grafting.

SUMMARY

Injuries to the larynx and trachea are rare. However, a high degree of suspicion is necessary for trauma patients with the right mechanism and examination findings, because early identification and treatment leads to better outcomes. Securing the airway is the first priority, with an awake tracheostomy being the ideal method in patients with displaced laryngeal fractures with or without substantial endolaryngeal injury. Early open reduction and internal fixation of displaced laryngeal cartilage fractures is recommended. Endolaryngeal injuries are managed through a laryngofissure or through existing cartilage fractures. The use of a laryngeal stent or keel can help prevent synechiae and laryngeal stenosis. Complete laryngotracheal separation is often quickly fatal because of loss of the airway in the field.

CLINICS CARE POINTS

- The key step in treatment of any laryngeal injury is the establishment of a secure airway.
- Early intervention (within 24–48 hours) is an important factor for improved patient outcomes (functional speech, swallowing, and airway patency).
- An awake tracheostomy is the airway of choice with grade II or higher laryngeal injuries.

REFERENCES

1. Jewett BS, Shockley WW, Rutledge R. External laryngeal trauma analysis of 392 patients. Arch Otolaryngol Head Neck Surg 1999;125(8):877–80.
2. Schaefer SD. The acute management of external laryngeal trauma. A 27-year experience. Arch Otolaryngol Head Neck Surg 1992;118(6):598–604.
3. Bent JP, Silver JR, Porubsky ES. Acute laryngeal trauma: a review of 77 patients. Otolaryngol Head Neck Surg 1993;109(3 Pt 1):441–9.
4. Verschueren DS, Bell RB, Bagheri SC, et al. Management of laryngo-tracheal injuries associated with craniomaxillofacial trauma. J Oral Maxillofac Surg 2006;64(2):203–14.
5. Lynch M. Repair of the traumatized larynx. Laryngoscope 1951;61(1):51–65.
6. Nahum AM. Immediate care of acute blunt laryngeal trauma. J Trauma 1969;9(2):112–25.
7. Trone TH, Schaefer SD, Carder HM. Blunt and penetrating laryngeal trauma: a 13-year review. Otolaryngol Head Neck Surg (1979) 1980;88(3):257–61.
8. Fuhrman GM, Stieg FH, Buerk CA. Blunt laryngeal trauma: classification and management protocol. J Trauma 1990;30(1):87–92.
9. Stassen NA, Hoth JJ, Scott MJ, et al. Laryngotracheal injuries: does injury mechanism matter? Am Surg 2004;70(6):522–5.
10. Shi J, Uyeda JW, Duran-Mendicuti A, et al. Multidetector CT of laryngeal injuries: principles of injury recognition. Radiographics 2019;39(3):879–92.
11. Randall DR, Rudmik L, Ball CG, et al. Airway management changes associated with rising radiologic incidence of external laryngotracheal injury. Can J Surg 2018;61(2):121–7.
12. Montgomery WW, Montgomery SK. Manual for use of Montgomery laryngeal, tracheal, and esophageal prostheses: update 1990. Ann Otol Rhinol Laryngol 1990;150(9_suppl):2–28.
13. Schaefer SD. Management of acute blunt and penetrating external laryngeal trauma. Laryngoscope 2014;124(1):233–44.

Printed and bound by CPI Group (UK) Ltd, Croydon, CR0 4YY

08/05/2025

01864697-0013